The Ginseng Book

The Ginseng Book

NATURE'S ANCIENT HEALER

Stephen Fulder, Ph.D.

Avery Publishing Group

Garden City Park, New York

The therapeutic procedures in this book are based on the training, personal experiences, and research of the author. Because each person and situation is unique, the author and publisher urge the reader to check with a qualified health professional before using any procedure where there is any question to appropriateness.

The publisher does not advocate the use of any particular diet or health program, but believes the information presented in this book should be available to the public.

Because there is always some risk involved, the author and publisher are not responsible for any adverse effects or consequences resulting from the use of any of the suggestions, preparations, or procedures in this book. Please do not use the book if you are unwilling to assume the risk. Feel free to consult with a physician or other qualified health professional. It is a sign of wisdom, not cowardice, to seek a second or third opinion.

Library of Congress Cataloging-in-Publication Data

Fulder, Stephen.
    The ginseng book : nature's ancient healer / Stephen Fulder.
      p. cm.
    Includes bibliographical references and index.
    ISBN 0-89529-720-5
    1. Ginseng—Therapeutic use. I. Title.
    RM666.G49F835 1996
    615'.323687—dc20   95-44105
                                            CIP

Printed in the United States of America

10 9 8 7 6 5 4 3 2

Contents

Acknowledgments

I would like to thank Joseph Needham for the use of his library and Helen Varley and Arthur Rashap for comments on the manuscript. Of course, I would also like to acknowledge the help of ginseng, without which this book would have taken much longer to write.

Preface

In 1972, I found myself in the midst of postdoctoral work at the National Institute for Medical Research in London. My subject was gerontology, or the study of the aging process. I was researching how it was that human cells become old and whether there was an aging clock, ticking away in their genetic apparatus—their DNA. I was able to watch human cells grow old, over time, in laboratory culture dishes. Purely by chance a report came to my notice that a strange Oriental medicinal plant, called ginseng, could prolong the life of such cells in culture. I had no idea what this substance was. So I went down to the Portobello Road, London, to see a friend of mine who had a store selling herbs, trinkets, and knickknacks. I asked him about it. He reverently took down a small wood box and carefully unwrapped some gnarled, twisted, and yet translucent red roots, among the strangest that I had ever seen. They are most valuable, I was told, and they have a subtle power to slow down the aging process.

My curiosity was piqued. I bought some, took them back to the laboratory, ground them up, extracted them with hot water, and added a small amount to my cultures. There resulted indeed a very clear difference. The cells that were already getting on in life and were slow to grow and reluctant to multiply seemed to renew their earlier shape and activity. I then did an experiment on myself and took some of the roots every day for a week. I felt a remarkable effect: a surge of energy and positivity that stayed with me for that week and another week afterwards. I seemed to be able to accomplish twice as much and needed less sleep.

The intriguing fact was that there was nothing at all in the entire world of Western medicine and Western drugs that could be regarded as an anti-aging remedy—nothing at all that was available to help old people to function better, be more active and energetic, and feel more alive. Ginseng seemed to me to be a wonderful and desperately needed remedy, strange though it was. I began to do serious research on ginseng with animals and in clinical studies with old people. More than that, I began to explore the world of traditional Oriental medicine that had given birth to such an exciting remedy. It led me into a completely different path in life, for to this day I have been researching and using safe natural remedies from the Eastern and Western herbal traditions. It also led me to write this book in order to tell ginseng's remarkable story.

At that time, ginseng was totally unknown in the West. Ginseng today is a household word. It is advertised on national television and is available in most drug stores. Health stores stock many different kinds and forms of it. The total sales of herbal products in 1995 in the USA is projected to be some $770 million, and of this, approximately $100 million will be ginseng. The public have forgotten that only a few years ago, ginseng was regarded as a mysterious and probably useless Oriental fad, known in America only to the Chinese of Chinatown and a few herbal experts.

But despite this extensive use today, there is still much

misunderstanding and ignorance about ginseng. Some think it is a kind of Oriental aphrodisiac, well tried and recommended by the ancient Chinese emperors; some think it is a stimulant that can enhance performance, like a strong cup of coffee; some think of it as a kind of storybook panacea, and perhaps because of this, others assume it is utter hyperbole. All of these views have some truth in them. But ginseng is much more than any of them, and to those that understand what it really is and how it can be used, it can be a real aid to vitality and well-being.

The purpose of this book is therefore not only to introduce ginseng to those who have never heard of it, but also to dispel the myth and the mystery, to show ginseng as it is—an important and effective new health remedy that can achieve results no modern drug can possibly achieve. To show ginseng in its full potential, it is not enough to look at it from the scientific perspective alone, nor only from the world of legends and traditions. It is necessary to search for the truth about ginseng in all the worlds—to journey to the East and examine the Oriental herbal tradition, the legends, the stories, and the current attitudes toward it; to explore the scientific research, which is now a huge body of literature; and finally to view it with the eyes of a modern herbal expert.

What we find is that ginseng is a subtle and yet powerful plant remedy that can help us in areas where a remedy is badly needed: in improving the quality of our energy and vitality and in helping us to resist more effectively the stresses and strains of life. It can help us overcome exhaustion and "burnout," convalescence and periods of special stress, and of course to arrive in old age skipping, not crawling.

Those who strive to go beyond
normal human limits will remain light
and strong, and although they grow
old in years they will remain
able-bodied and flourishing . . .

—*The Yellow Emperors*
Book of Internal Medicine

CHAPTER 1

A Natural
Health Enhancer

O f all the multitude of plant medicines known, ginseng is surely one of the most interesting. No other plant is used so widely in the Orient for so many health purposes. A look at the nature of the plant, its role in ancient medicine, and the difference between tradition and myth may help us reach an understanding of how ginseng fits into modern health promotion and maintenance.

What makes ginseng unique? For thousands of years, it has been regarded as a universally beneficial remedy. Its full name, *Panax ginseng*, illustrates this, for Panax, like panacea, comes from the Greek word for "all healing." In fact, the Chinese, whose traditional medicine is without doubt one of the most sophisticated medical systems known, do not even believe in the notion of a "cure-all." They are concerned with "health" rather than "healing," regard ginseng as having extraordinary powers in promoting well-being, and rely heavily on it as an essential tonic and restorative. It is also a regular ingredient that serves as a "booster" in the complex array of medicinal plant mixtures used for the direct treatment of serious diseases.

We can understand this approach a little better if we consider the Chinese philosophy of the Tao, literally, "the way." It is the incomprehensible flow of energy of the cosmos which finds its temporary expression in the materials of nature. Man is also made of these materials, and he will be healthy if he achieves harmony with the Tao, the essence of the world. Ginseng is believed to contain all the elements necessary to adjust the body of man in tune with nature. If man were in greater alignment with nature he would have more of its strength and energy, therefore it could have a profound effect on health if used wisely.

Ginseng also is the plant used most widely to combat some of the degenerative conditions and loss of vitality that accompany aging, and, not surprisingly, a special reverence for it has developed over the centuries. Ginseng represents a beneficial aspect of nature, which is why it is treated as such a great gift. It is embodied in many stories and legends; in fact, probably no other plant has such an extensive mythology.

Ginseng is uniquely important because it is most typical of traditional Oriental medicine. If we can unravel some of its subtleties it will tell us about the medical system that gave it prominence.

THE GINSENG PLANT

Panax ginseng is the botanical name given to the Asian ginseng plant by the botanist and explorer Carl Anton Meyer. It belongs to the small family called the *Araliaceae*, which includes, among others, Indian root, sarsaparilla, and ivy. For such a famous plant, it looks remarkably humble. It has arrays of five saw-toothed leaves atop a long, straight stalk, which may be about 8 to 30 inches tall, depending on age. Older plants may have two or more of these stalks. Its pale green flowers begin to appear only when the plant is two or three years old. These produce bright red berries, well-liked by people and birds. The latter spread the seeds, which are the size of small lentils.

The medicinal part of ginseng is the thick, fleshy root. It is somewhat like a carrot but yellow, not orange. It has many tendrils and rootlets and may sometimes be branched, curled, or bent. At the top of the root is a crinkled "neck," actually a short underground stem that bears the buds for each season's growth. The fresh root tastes somewhat bitter, with a hint of aromatic sweetness.

Ginseng is a deciduous perennial; that is, the above-ground foliage dies off every autumn and the root lies under the cold winter ground until April or May, when one or more buds on the neck sprout new stems. The flowers spread in June, the seeds ripen in August, and the foliage yellows and dies by October, leaving the root ready for another winter dormancy. Each annual cycle leaves a wrinkle on the neck above the root, an easy guide to the age of the plant.

Asian ginseng once grew naturally in the high temperate forests of China, Korea, and the Eastern part of the former USSR, but it is now virtually extinct in its wild state. However, cultivation has spread the domesticated ginseng to many other areas in Eastern Asia. Although the Chinese undoubtedly value the wild ginseng above perhaps any other plant, they regard even the cultivated variety as probably their most important medicine.

Manchuria is the traditional home of the most expensive and highest quality wild ginseng. The Manchurians boast that "the weeds of their country are the choice drugs of the Chinese." It is often mentioned that one Chinese emperor set out to war in order to capture ginseng-growing land,

and it is certainly true that in 1709 the Emperor sent ten thousand Tartars to search for ginseng, ordering that each soldier should give him two catties (about two and a half pounds) of the best and sell the rest for its weight in silver.

The closest cousin to Asian ginseng is the native species of North America, described botanically as *Panax quinquefolium*. It looks like a compact version of Asian ginseng and is famous as a medicine among the North American Indians. Such close resemblances are common between Chinese species of flora and fauna, including the medicinal plants, and those on the American side of the Pacific. *Panax quinquefolium* also grows naturally in the Himalayas and is cultivated in China.

Other Panax species are used in traditional medicine, but none has the same reputation. *Panax pseudoginseng* has a short fat root and seven leaves, more narrow than those of ginseng, leading to its Chinese name "jen-seng San-ch'i" (three seven ginseng). It grows in China, especially in Yunnan, and there is a Japanese variety. Then there are a few Himalayan relatives scattered throughout the forests of Nepal, Sikkim, Bhutan, Tibet, and Assam. One plant— the mandrake—has been mistakenly called a relative. It has a man-shaped root like ginseng, but botanically it is not even distantly related, and medicinally it will knock you down, not pick you up.

HISTORY AND LEGEND

In ancient China, the general opinion was that ginseng was the prince of plants. Emperor Shen Nung, the most famous Chinese herbalist and one of the founders of Chinese traditional medicine, put forward a classification of herbs that is recorded in the *Shen Nung Pen Tshao Ching*, the *Pharmacopoeia of the Heavenly Husbandman*, printed in the second century BC. Several hundred herbs were listed. Ginseng is at the top of the list of those agents that are beneficial yet harmless.

The Chinese sometimes kept ginseng in lead-lined boxes, carefully wrapped in silk and tissue paper, believing that it gave off certain "life-giving radiations" that might be lost in an ordinary container. Such radiations are in fact unlikely, but the tradition illustrates the reverential and almost sacramental treatment given to the herb.

This respect is reflected in the fabulous prices that were paid for the wild root during imperial times. An old wild root, cured properly and of the best quality, would fetch much more than its weight in gold, giving rise to the sarcastic Manchurian epithet: "Eat ginseng and ruin yourself."

The word *ginseng* is derived from the words jen shen, which means "a crystallization of the essence of the earth (shen) in the form of a man (jen)" or more simply, "man root." The same word also means "like the constellation of Orion," which is traditionally shaped like a man. It is also the constellation that has astrological influence over ginseng. Other names of ginseng are: blood-like (hsueh shen), human bridle (jen hsien), devil cover (kuei kai), magical herb (shen tshao), and a more literal name, "the regenerating elixir that banishes wrinkles from the face" (tson mien huntan). The Koreans call the herb Korean phoenix (poughwang). The Japanese name is more prosaic: Korean carrot.

It is believed that the plant's power to cure a certain part of the body is reflected in some ways in its form. Thus, since a ginseng root is shaped like a man, it was believed to have great curative powers for the whole body, particularly the restoration of male potency. Such a wild root will still fetch thousands of dollars among Chinese people living overseas (who are more likely than those living in mainland China to be able to afford it). This is also the cost of a treatment with wild ginseng in Korea today, for those lucky enough to find a traditional practitioner who possesses such a rarity.

China is not the only place where ginseng has been used since ancient times. The Vedas are ancient Indian scriptures reflecting an oral teaching that may be five thousand years old. The Atherva Veda has many hymns describing ways to attain health and fulfillment. One hymn describes ginseng as "the root which is dug from the earth and which strengthens the nerves." It continues: "the strength of the horse, the mule, the goat, the ram, moreover the strength of the bull it bestows on him. This herb will make thee so full of lusty strength that thou shalt, when excited, exhale heat as a thing on fire."

The hymn then describes the herb as "brother of Soma." Soma is the legendary life-giving plant of India, an elixir that was worshipped and offered in sacrifices. If ginseng is the brother of Soma, it must also have appeared to have unearthly power. However, ginseng is not a feature of the Ayurvedic medical system, which developed out of the Vedas, perhaps because it became unavailable in India.

A medicinal plant as important as ginseng may be more than just a medicine to the people who use it. It is sometimes seen as a veritable gift from benign divine powers. Extensive ritual can surround the gathering, planting, storing, preparing, and consuming of the root, and the many legends have given rise to many names. One story describes how the village of Shantan, in Shensi province, was troubled for many nights by a groaning and wailing somewhere behind the village. Although much afraid of this strange occurrence, the villagers organized an expedition one night to discover the source of the unearthly cries. They took torches and wooden sticks and eventually localized the sound to a large bush about a mile away. When they dug up the bush and revealed its huge root, the shape and size of a man, the crying stopped. From this the root became known as "spirit of the earth" (ti ching).

Wherever it grows, ginseng has given rise to its own myths. In Korea, it is related how an ailing man was being looked after devotedly by his son and grandson, both very poor. One night the grandson couldn't sleep. The candle kept blowing out. He was suddenly aware that there was no wind to blow out the candle so there must be a spirit presence in the room. The boy took a needle and thread, and the next time he felt the presence of the spirit he plunged the needle in that direction. The needle disappeared, but the boy followed the thread and eventually found the needle stuck in the ground at the base of a wild ginseng plant. He took the plant and brewed a decoction for his grandfather, who recovered. Thus the spirit of the ginseng plant rewarded the boy for his selfless devotion.

There are many more myths and rituals, some of which will be related in discussions of the way ginseng is collected, cultivated, cured, and consumed. The essence of the legends is that ginseng has an almost supernatural power for the good of man. But its power is not just legendary. As will become clear in subsequent chapters, no other plant has been the subject of such extensive scientific research yielding such controversial conclusions. Finally, it will become strikingly obvious that there is no other medicinal plant that is so widely respected in one half of the world and so misunderstood in the other half.

CHAPTER 2

The Basis of
Herbal Medicine

Those who scorn ginseng and other herbal remedies as acquiring their value purely from folklore and superstitition clearly have no insight into the complex and rational basis of Oriental medicine. In fact, traditional Western medicine's official view of herbal remedies has shifted from positive to negative and now back again as the West has finally begun to examine herbal medicine with a more open mind, and to assess it through valid scientific methods.

Plants are essential to life. Virtually all the food we eat is from the plant kingdom or from animals who eat plants. Plants also enhance health, and the number of different types used as medicines is even greater than the number used for food. Several thousand years before Christ, traditional Indian medicine held that not a single plant on earth is useless. As it says in the Vedas, the sacred Sanskrit texts that describe the ancient system:

All the many herbs in which the human physicians find a remedy,

Like mothers assembled let them yield milk
Unto man, for freedom from harm.

Many plants, such as Digitalis, Rauwolfia, Datura, and
Ephedra, are used exclusively for medicines; others—for
example, garlic, mint, coffee, banana, caraway, and licorice—
are both food and medicine. In Chinese and Western natural
medicine, there is little difference between a food and a
medicine. The path to health involves all the substances
consumed by and connected to the human organism.

THE WESTERN VIEW OF TRADITIONAL MEDICINE

As might be expected, the view of herbal remedies held by
practitioners of traditional medicine is very different from
that held by most conventional doctors. Dr. Williams, working in China at the turn of the twentieth century, wrote
cynically about Chinese traditional medicine: "Anything indeed that is thoroughly disgusting in the three kingdoms of
Nature is considered good enough for medicinal use."

In fact, conventional medicine essentially rid itself of traditional plant remedies during the early part of this century,
describing them as unproven and uncertain concoctions perhaps fit for grandmothers to dispense but not doctors. Almost none are left in any official Western pharmacopeia, or
list of acceptable drugs. They were discarded without ever
being tested to see whether they could in fact achieve the
results that traditional practitioners and their patients
claimed for them. Plants were banished by the fashion for
chemicals, the emerging pharmaceutical industry, and the
creed of scientific medicine rather than by evidence of inef-
fectiveness. Modern medicine thereby limited its options to
stronger chemical drugs. Only now, after many years of
concern and alarm at the pervasive side effects of such drugs,

is there a renewed interest in those mild plant remedies and medicinal foods that were left by the wayside. Such plants as aloes, comfrey, garlic, feverfew, camomile, or licorice are slowly beginning to be investigated again.

The medicinal resources in the plant world are enormous, most of them completely unknown to science. It is reliably estimated that science has investigated for medicinal activity less than one percent of plant species. Chinese traditional medicine, in contrast, has developed through thousands of years of experience, observation, and experiment. It knows which plants to use, for what purposes, how and when to use them, in what combinations, and for which types of person.

THE ESSENCE OF HEALTH

We can return to the second century B.C. and the *Pharmacopoeia of the Heavenly Husbandmen* to find an interesting clue to the way ginseng and other herbs have been used in China. It states that ginseng is a "tonic to the five viscera, quieting the animal spirits, strengthening the soul, allaying fear, expelling evil effluvia, brightening the eyes, opening the heart, benefiting the understanding, and if taken for some time, it will invigorate the body and prolong life."

More modern Eastern pharmacopeias echo this earliest record. They state that ginseng alleviates tiredness, headaches, exhaustion, amnesia, and the debilitating effects of old age, and they confirm that it is a useful adjunct in the treatment of tuberculosis, diabetes, and diseases of the heart, kidneys, and nervous and circulatory systems. It is said to prevent declining potency in older men. A recent Chinese text, for example, states that it is used for anyone with general weakness, including "those with signs of anemia, lack of appetite, shortness of breath accompanied by perspiration, nervousness, forgetfulness, thirst, lack of strength, and lack of sexual desire." In other words, though it is not a cure for specific diseases, it is regarded as a powerful restorative agent, which has effects that are not limited to any organ or tissue but are spread throughout the body.

Its ability to increase general vitality is what makes it so precious in the eyes of the Chinese, for they regard vitality as the essence of health. This is why it is one of the most important Chinese medicines. But the breadth of Eastern claims for ginseng has confused Westerners. Asian herbalists saw that ginseng increased vitality and heat, making available an added source of energy to diverse organs and thus helping in a large variety of health problems. Westerners wrongly assumed that any one remedy said to assist in so many conditions must be a panacea, and gave it the name Panax. Since a panacea is an ultimate consumer product, advertisers took up the message and touted it as a cure for every disease imaginable. Ginseng, to Asians an essential tool for maintaining and improving health, became to Westerners a cure-all, therefore a joke.

PRINCIPLES AND PRACTICES OF CHINESE TRADITIONAL MEDICINE

Eastern medicine does not even have the concept of a "cure-all." It is more concerned with "all-health." Chinese traditional medicine is probably the most complicated and esoteric medical system known, little of which is properly understood in the West. It is helpful to take a brief look at some key principles of traditional Eastern medicine.

The Goal of Maintaining Peak Condition

Western medicine regards the powerful drugs as the mainstay of treatment and the mild drugs as accessories of little significance. Chinese medicine takes exactly the opposite approach. The mildest herbs are the most important and of the first rank, while the really powerful herbs are the last-resort drugs to be used only when the others fail. Those that have a mild effect and are not harmful, even in large doses, are called "kingly," for example, ginseng, licorice, and jujube (Chinese dates). The second group, which are more powerful and rather more toxic, are called "ministerial." The lowest group, called merely "servant," are the highly powerful and dangerous herbs, including aconite (wolfsbane) and hellebore.

Underlying this approach to herbal pharmacology is the most basic principle of Chinese traditional medicine, which is the attempt to maintain the body in peak condition. If the body is healthy, it will automatically be more resistant to disease, just as a car that is tuned and serviced will be much less likely to have a serious breakdown. Therefore the task of traditional practitioners is primarily to ensure the continuing health of the people they look after and only secondarily to treat diseases. A Chinese doctor used to be paid by his patients only when they were in good health. When they became ill the doctor was not paid, because he had failed to keep his patient healthy. It is fair to say that while the focus of traditional medicine is on health, the focus of conventional medicine is on sickness. We can now see why the mild herbs, especially ginseng, are the "kingly" ones. They are the primary weapon of practitioners in health maintenance.

Yin and Yang

Superimposed on the fundamental concept just discussed are complex instructions relating different herbs to different kinds of disturbances in body functions. The body, like all of nature, consists of active, male, expanding, burning, or "yang" qualities and passive, female, contracting, conserving, or "yin" qualities. For health, these qualities must be in an equilibrium that takes into account the person's constitutional type and the yin and yang forces in foods, the weather, and the general environment. Ginseng is extremely yang. Its effect is to burn up wastes and increase the flow of energy in an organ system, so it is taken when organ systems are too yin and sluggish.

The energizing yang nature of ginseng is well understood by Asian practitioners, and it is their guide to when and how to take this herb. Its special virtue is to ward off tiredness, exhaustion, convalescence, and the effects of advanced age—states of health where energy is depleted and the body has slowed down. It is, by the same token, not very effective for anyone who is vital, young, energetic, and alert.

Achieving a Harmony of Elements

Another key principle of Chinese medicine lies in the five elements: wood, fire, earth, metal, and water, similar to the early Greek elements of earth, air, fire, and water. These are poetic metaphors that refer to the texture and constitution of natural forces or processes. For example, earth implies solidity, and fire, activity. Health requires a proper relationship between the elements in the body and those in the external world. Ginseng, the root of man, is described as benefiting and harmonizing all the elements. However, Asian ginseng is regarded as predominantly a heating remedy, beneficial in conditions where the body is cold or watery, which makes it susceptible to cold and damp diseases such as those of the joints. For this reason it is understood that:

- Ginseng is best used to increase health and prevent disease in autumn and winter, not summer.

- Ginseng helps prevent and treat "cold" diseases, including those of poor or inadequate circulation, elimination or digestion, weakness, metabolism, and sexual activity.

- Ginseng is better used in colder climates.

- Ginseng will be arousing, stimulating, or "heating" to the brain.

Combining Remedies

Traditionally, an Oriental remedy is rarely used alone. The Chinese have developed a wonderfully sophisticated method of building combinations of plants that help each other, and three-fourths of all Chinese medicines contain more than four ingredients. If a strong remedy, such as *Rehmannia glutinosa,* is used to stimulate an organ—say the kidney—it is combined with others, such as *Alisma plantago* (water plantain), to quench or disperse the heat created by Rehmannia's action, in other words, to remove waste and protect the organ while treating it. If Ephedra (ephedrine, a bronchodilator) is given to promote sweating and clear out a cough and cold, cinnamon may be added to help the circulation and apricot seed to promote the coughing up of phlegm, which Ephreda would otherwise prevent. Licorice would be added to combine all the ingredients, remove poisons, and protect the stomach.

Ginseng is one of the most frequently used Oriental remedies. It is present in more than a quarter of all classical prescriptions, a majority of which are adjustive, preventive, and restorative, or "kingly," as opposed to those that are more directly curative. It is also a component of quite a few mixtures for more serious diseases, such as those of the circulation or nervous system, although not usually as the curative backbone of the recipe. It is more likely to be there to support the patient's energy and vitality while other plants work directly against the disorder.

A classical authority, Chieh-pin Chang, published a book in AD 960 listing more than 500 formulas containing ginseng, covering nearly every type of disease. Some examples follow.

A typical general tonic, developed by Li Shih Chen, China's most famous herbalist of the seventeenth century, is:

Ginseng extract	2 parts
Root of *Atractylis lancea*	2 parts
"Fou ling" (*Pachyma cocos*)	2 parts
Licorice (*Glycyrrhiza uralensis*)	1 part
Ginger	1 part
Red Jujube dates (*Zizyphus jujube*)	1 part

The "Vital Essence" formula, said to build the male hormones and increase virility and energy, includes:

Lycium fruits (*Lycium chinensis*)	2 parts
Schizandra chinensis	2 parts
Ginseng	1 part
Deer Antler	1 part

Here's a typical recovery tonic to restore health quickly after a disease, increase energy, get rid of poisons, and improve metabolism:

Ginseng	3 parts
Wild Asparagus root (*Asparagus licidus*)	5 parts
Schizandra chinensis berries	5 parts

Rehmannia glutinosa	2 parts
Ligusticum lucidum	2 parts
Tree Peony	2 parts
Bitter Orange Peel (*citrus aurantium*)	1 part
Licorice (*Glycyrrhiza uralensis*)	1 part

The other components of a mixture can augment the effects of ginseng in subtle and remarkable ways. For example, licorice will direct the action of ginseng to the metabolism and strengthen immunity. *Cimifuga heracleifolia* will focus it on the lungs, and Poria cocos directs ginseng to the kidneys. Ginger is described as a servant that helps ginseng warm and strengthen the body, and orange peel spreads its effects evenly throughout the body.

THE SPECIFIC USES OF GINSENG

During its long history of use, ginseng has earned the reputation of having a variety of applications. The discussions below review some of the most important and common uses of this miraculous root.

Maintaining and Restoring Strength and Stamina

All countries where ginseng is used traditionally hold that it is a stimulant and that it can increase the resistance of the body. The sick take it to restore strength. Chinese soldiers carry it into battle to prevent the effects of stress and shock if they are wounded and sustain them until they can be brought to the field hospital. Soldiers use it as a stimulant while on sentry duty, and it is recorded that the North Vietnamese used it extensively in the recent war.

After a series of experiments at their cosmodrome, Soviet experts in space medicine concluded that ginseng was a better stimulant or tonic for their cosmonauts than the amphetamines used by American astronauts. It increased alertness and performance more successfully, without preventing proper sleep or producing hangovers. Cosmonauts took ginseng and related plants with them on space missions in the 1970s.

Soviet sportsmen found it similarly useful. After a long series of trials, particularly at the Lesgraft Institute of Physical Culture and Sports, the director, Professor Anton Korobov, concluded that the action of ginseng-like plants should be "aimed at accelerating the restorative processes after intensive activity and increasing the body's resistance to unfavorable external influence." The result was that Soviet sportsmen were officially instructed by the sports ministry to take ginseng or a Soviet relative, Eleutherococcus, to help overcome exhaustion and stress during training. They also use them in sports events, including the Olympics, to gain access to every last ounce of energy.

The stimulant action of ginseng is graphically described by Father Jartoux, the French priest who brought it to the notice of the Royal Society of London in 1714. While he was surveying the Chinese border with Korea, a local Mandarin gave him some ginseng. "In an Hour after I found my Pulse much fuller and quicker, I had an Appetite, and found myself much more vigorous and could bear Labour much better and easier than before," he wrote. Later, he rode with the Chinese emperor until he was so exhausted that he could hardly keep from falling off his horse. The emperor gave him half a root of ginseng, which he chewed, whereupon he forgot all about his fatigue and carried on full of energy.

The plant is believed capable of saving the lives of seriously ill patients by giving them the energy, vitality, and stamina to fight their disease. The Chinese have described many cases in which the sick have been near death, when administration of good quality ginseng root revived them sufficiently to deal with business matters. It is a common practice in China to give ginseng to someone on his deathbed to provide him with the strength to receive his family and arrange his affairs. As Dr. Porter Smith noticed: "Several cases in which life would seem to have been at least prolonged by taking doses of the drug so as to allow intelligent disposal of property indicate that some positive efficacy of a sustaining character does really exist in this species."

Other non-Asians have made similar comments. For example, Dr. Whittie, a Fellow of the Royal College of Physicians in the seventeenth century, was given some ginseng, which he used on a patient who was:

> much emaciated, and reduced into a perfect Skeleton, a meer Bag of Bones, by a long Hectic Feaver, joyned with an Ulcer of the Lungs; being despaired of by all Friends, I was resolved to try what the Tincture of This Root could doe, which I gave every morning in Red Cows Milk, warm from her Duggs. And I found his Flesh to come again like that of a Child, and his lost Appetite restored, and his natural Ruddy Complexion revived in his Cheeks to the Amazement of his desponding Relations, that he was called 'Lazarus the Second.'

Maintaining Sexual Strength and Virility

Ginseng has also earned a reputation as an aphrodisiac (a drug that stimulates sexual desire). In fact, the *Encyclopaedia Britannica* uses ginseng as an example of a "genuine" aphrodisiac.

There are many records of its use by Chinese Emperors and their courts to maintain the required Imperial virility, a symbol of the health of the Empire. Many of the Asian tonic remedies are concerned with the maintenance of sexual energy, partly because Eastern cultures see it as a crucial sign of overall good health. Ginseng is often combined for this purpose with such other herbs and exotic materials as sea horses, deer horn, and various animal organ extracts. Not unexpectedly, this has caught the imagination of Westerners. Ginseng is certainly found in sex shops and occasionally turns up as the subject of waggish comment in the media. This has led most of the public to view ginseng as "some kind of aphrodisiac." The Chinese do not claim that it is an aphrodisiac, a specific sexual stimulant. Indeed, even the extent of its use for this purpose in Asia is uncertain. While the Emperors are known to have consumed much ginseng at court, they probably took it as a general tonic to improve their overall vitality rather than as an aphrodisiac per se. It may be that its reputation as such owes more to the fancy of European observers at the Imperial court than to fact.

A somewhat similar mistake may have been made in describing it as an aphrodisiac as in describing it as a panacea. The quite remarkable property of ginseng is to increase deep vitality and energy. One of the results of improving access to this energy may well be increased sexual virility. Another frequent result may be increased memory and mental function. But it cannot be called a memory drug or an aphrodisiac because of its positive effects on overall human performance, just as it cannot be described as a cure-all because of its positive effects on overall health.

On the other hand, ginseng is used widely to combat impotence, especially the decline in virility which occurs with age. Travellers to Asia from Marco Polo on have also been impressed by the virility of elderly Chinese people, and the Chinese themselves readily admit that the use of ginseng is partly responsible.

Protecting Against the Diseases of Old Age

The herbal tradition of ginseng states explicitly that the more it is taken, the more long-term benefits can be obtained. It is recommended that everyone who can afford it should take a course of ginseng every year. The effect is cumulative, and regular use, it is said, not only increases health and vitality but prolongs life. Old people are advised to take some every day to extend their life span and enhance protection from the diseases of old age. If it could be authenticated that it is really a "regenerative elixir that banishes wrinkles from the face," it would be the first medicine or drug to be specifically useful for the aged. A subsequent chapter will be devoted to this intriguing possibility.

Other Eastern countries that use ginseng in traditional ways ascribe almost identical properties to it. The *Materia Indica* of 1826, for example, states that ginseng "nourishes and strengthens the body, stops vomiting, clears the judgment, removes hypochondrias and all nervous affectations, and in a word, gives vigorous tone to the body even in old age."

When ginseng was first brought to Europe its special ability to improve vigor in the aged and thus, perhaps, to increase longevity was particularly noted. As one seventeenth-century English doctor wrote: "Public Fame saith, that the Popes of Rome, who are chosen to that Office when they are very Old, doe make great use of this Root, to preserve their Radical Moysture and natural Heat, that so they may the longer enjoy their Comfortable Preferments."

While William Byrd, a Fellow of the Royal Society and author, noted that though it did not appear to be useful in "Feats of Love," it gives "uncommon Warmth and Vigor to the Blood and frisks the Spirit, beyond any other Cordial . . . it will make a Man live a great while, and very well while he does live. And what is more, it will even make Old Age amicable, by rendering it lively, chearful and good-humour'd . . ."

AN AMERICAN COUSIN

American ginseng, *Panax quinquefolium*, is exported in large quantities to Asia. It is botanically close to Asian ginseng and is often regarded as its equivalent, so the word ginseng usually covers both without differentiation. This confusion of species, however, has damaged ginseng's reputation, for the august Smithsonian Institute tested the American ginseng, and finding it ineffective as a stimulant declared that all ginseng is worthless. But are they equivalent? Are the traditional claims made for it the same as those for Asian ginseng?

Panax quinquefolium is regarded by its native North American discoverers much as Asians do their ginseng, but with less hyperbole and veneration. They do not regard it as the chief of their medicines but describe it as an aid to digestion and appetite and a help for cramps and menstrual problems. The Creeks, for example, drank an infusion of the root for exhaustion, breathlessness, and croup. Other tribes describe it as a supportive aid for the wounded. Cherokees, much like Asians, describe their ginseng as "the little man" and acknowledge it as a tonic. Clearly, they all understand its support for energy and metabolism but do not use it as a stimulant or rejuvenating medicine.

In China, where both roots are available, the traditional view is that American ginseng is yin while Asian ginseng is yang. It improves the function of the organs by balancing the flow of their metabolism rather than speeding it up, so it is taken to improve health, energy, and resistance. Interestingly, its predominantly yin "female" quality makes it more suitable for women, whereas Asian ginseng is more suitable for men. Similarly, it is used in preference to Asian ginseng in hot climates or during summer months. As it is a sedative rather than stimulating tonic, it is used by people who need vitality but are already constitutionally yang, that is, active, agitated, nervous, or hot. For such people, the Asian root might create excessive stimulation while the American root could help build their strength and allow proper rest.

Why is it then that American ginseng is appreciated so much in China and the Orient, but in America itself and other Western countries, only the Asian ginseng is used? The answer is that in the West, where people are more interested in getting the most out of life, ginseng is taken as a short-term tonic to aid vitality and energy and to increase performance. Therefore the "yang" stimulatory action of the Asian species is appreciated. The Chinese, on the other hand, take ginseng rather more for the purposes of achieving inner balance and aging well. In this case American and Asian ginseng are of equivalent value, each being used by people of different constitutions at different times. For example, a young Chinese woman who is thin, active, fit, energetic, well motivated, and living in a warm climate would prefer to take the more yin *Panax quinquefolium* in order to balance and economize on her energy and metabolism. On the other hand, her grandmother, who is getting quite old and is slow and sometimes tired and weak, would value the Asian ginseng for its warming, energizing power.

Of the other ginseng species only san-ch'i ginseng, *Panax pseudoginseng var. notoginseng,* is found much in traditional medicine. It is a weak tonic whose main use is to disperse unwanted blood in bruises, swellings, internal bleeding, and irregular menstruation. Himalayan tribes and Indian doctors use the Himalayan relatives of ginseng as minor medicines in cases of poor appetite and weak digestion.

CHINESE MEDICINE TODAY

Traditional medicine in China is not an archaic code of instructions present only in old books. It is a living system used today in a unique synthesis with conventional medicine. For example, in the teaching hospitals of Peking, surgery is carried out in the Western manner with highly advanced equipment, but the anesthetist may use acupuncture instead of conventional anesthetics, and herbal preparations are used for preoperative and postoperative treatment. Ginseng is often present in these preparations to increase the patient's resistance, protect the system against shock during the operation, and increase vitality during postoperative recovery.

Western medicine came to China during the last century. Hospitals and clinics were built and traditional medicine suppressed. However, during the chaos of the revolutionary period when modern medicines became unavailable, traditional medicine proved invaluable; afterwards it was reinstated alongside Western medicine. Rural health workers, the famous "barefoot doctors," taught sanitation and gave vaccinations in the villages, while traditional practitioners gave acupuncture treatment, herbs, and massage.

Traditional medicine then spread to the cities, where it is now studied at research institutes. In this way the Chinese hope to extract the best from four thousand years of experience in herbal medicine and acupuncture. The Chinese have not succeeded in understanding ancient principles in scientific terms. However, they have proved that traditional medicine works, whether or not it conforms to the current scientific theories. Chinese herbal medicine is impressive when judged with a "proof of the pudding" attitude. As an eminent pharmacologist, Dr. Louis Lasagna, remarked on a visit to China: "We may look forward to a whole range of new drugs of enormous potential for medicine in general." Ginseng is the first of these.

CHAPTER 3

From Cultivation
to Purchase

G inseng is now available in markets worldwide. Yet, it is no longer found abun-
dantly in the wild, is difficult to grow, and
varies widely in its quality, effects, and price, depending
not only on country of origin and type of plant but on
different methods of cultivation and preparation for use.

Among the many names given to ginseng is "The Root
that Hides from Man." This is meant literally, for the root
prefers a habitat deep within thick forest, in moist, rich,
and undisturbed soil. It sometimes favors specific trees as
neighbors, as this Korean song shows:

> The branches which grow from my stalks are
> three in number, and the leaves are five by five,
> The back part of the leaves is turned to the sky,
> and the upper side downwards,
> Whoever would find me must look for the Kia
> tree.

Finding wild ginseng was always so difficult that

searchers could do little else but pray to the spirits that guard it to favor their quest. In Korea, a team of wild ginseng gatherers would keep chaste and pure for a week before an expedition, praying continuously to their guardian deity. The team was always a group of ten senior villagers led by "The Man." They used a secret sign language during their quest and refrained from talking, for they were fearful of incurring the displeasure of nature spirits guarding the ginseng.

In China it is related how searchers took advantage of the glow that sometimes came from the leaves of the ginseng plant at night. The glow would go out if anyone approached, so a searcher would shoot an arrow at it and come back in daylight to look for the arrow and pull the plant. The glow has led to some extravagant theories concerning supposed radiations from ginseng. The cause is more likely to be glow-worms or moonlight reflected from the leaves.

Most of the gathering of wild ginseng in Manchuria used to be done on behalf of the Emperor, so the common people had to try poaching or make do with inferior cultivated or imported roots. A few plants still grow wild in Manchuria, the Ussuri region of the former USSR, and Korea, but extensive picking and the felling of forests have largely dried up supplies of the wild root in the East. No more than a kilo or two of genuine wild roots are dug every year in the whole of Asia, and these roots are likely to fetch thousands of dollars each when they find their way to the market. There is still sufficient wild American ginseng, *Panax quinquefolium*, to yield about 100,000 pounds a year. However, it has now been declared an endangered species and its export is regulated by the government.

Most of the ginseng now sold worldwide is not gathered in the wild. Instead, it is painstakingly cultivated, harvested, and prepared for market.

THE CULTIVATION OF GINSENG

The earliest ginseng plantations were in southeast Manchuria and North Korea, where cultivation is still carried out, although the product is entirely for home consumption. Major cultivation areas have developed in China, South Korea, Japan, and the former USSR. United States consular reports describe how the Russians started ginseng plantations in South Siberia with $120 million worth of young plants taken home from North Korea in the aftermath of the war. The Russians have wound down ginseng cultivation in the last 25 years in favor of other Araliaceous plants (as will be described later in this chapter).

Cultivation in Asia is big business, earning South Korea, for example, about $100 million annually. Yet it is still carried out with ceremony and elaborate preparation. Prayers are said before sowing the seeds into specially prepared germination beds in the autumn, a year after they are collected. The seeds need to lie dormant during the intermediate year, or more precisely the cold of an intermediate winter, to get ready for germination, and then they need the second winter to complete dormancy. They germinate in the spring and grow one year in their seed beds, after which they are usually transplanted to new beds with appropriate spacing. In Asia they may be transplanted at least once more before harvest, which will be in the autumn of the fourth, fifth, or sixth year, when the above-ground parts are yellow and dying off and the root has collected the most nutrients.

Ginseng cultivation requires well drained, clay-based, loamy soil containing organic matter such as leaf mold. Preferably, the field should face north and slope gently. The plant does not need a great deal of fertilization or manuring as it is slow-growing, but the earth should be slightly acid (pH 5.5). Shade, which is required to mimic the natural deep forest growing conditions, is provided in Asia by rolls of straw matting spread on frames over the bed. Korean research has shown that the plant grows best with shading that only lets through 20 percent of the light. The beds should be heavily mulched with leaf litter or other materials such as straw.

Ginseng is difficult to grow because of all the pests and diseases, especially fungi, that affect it in the close confines of intensive cultivation. Traditional methods, developed over 400 years in Asia, include protecting the plant by frequent transplanting to fresh beds and by using beds for growing ginseng that have had no ginseng growing on them for 12 years. This is not practical today, given the considerable pressure to grow ginseng in ever-greater quantities on an ever-diminishing supply of suitable land. The last few years have seen up to a third of the Asian ginseng crop affected by disease. Farmers have had to respond by extensive spraying, so that today cultivated Asian ginseng, though cheaper than before, may be laden with pesticides and fungicides.

Against this background, there is the cultivation in North America of 800,000 pounds of American ginseng (Panax quinquefolium) every year. Japan grows about the same amount of Asian ginseng, South Korea about three million pounds, and China about two-and-a-half million. American ginseng today is grown with a high level of agrotechnical expertise even though most is grown by family farmers who have switched from milk or potato production. Plastic shade net is used, and in contrast to Asia, the farms are mechanized. The roots are not transplanted during growth although they may be thinned, and disease is dealt with by extensive spraying with agrochemicals. This is another reason why Asian countries, under pressure to compete, are phasing out their traditional organic methods in favor of such modern agricultural methods.

THE PREPARATION OF GINSENG FOR MARKET

The ginseng root that is available in shops is never fresh. It has undergone an elaborate process of curing and drying that preserves the essential medicinal components and allows the root to be kept for years without decay or decline in potency. The dried root is hard and has a stronger, more aromatic and bittersweet taste than fresh root.

After the root is carefully dug from the earth, the fine outer tendrils are removed and it is washed. Some roots are steam cured by a process that turns them deep red and makes them remarkably translucent (red ginseng). Steaming is intended to preserve the root more effectively, the proof of which is provided by a red root placed in the Royal Storehouse of Shosin in Nara, Japan, in AD 756 by the Buddhist priest Kan-Jin. It is still in good condition, and laboratory analysis has demonstrated that it contains all the expected chemical constituents. Roots that are not steamed are yellow and opaque (white ginseng). Slow drying in a sequence of warm rooms at different temperatures for some months finally preserves and hardens the root and makes it ready for consumption.

THE PRICING OF GINSENG

The quality of the ginseng root varies considerably. This is to some extent reflected in the price, which is set by world demand. Of first quality is the wild Asian ginseng, hugely expensive and never seen outside Asia. Next in price is some old cultivated Asiatic ginseng, such as Chinese "tassel" ginseng. Then comes the majority of cultivated roots, whose price and quality vary with age. Asian red ginseng is usually of higher quality than the so-called white (actually yellow) because only the older and better roots are selected for the special steam process. Poorer quality roots tend to develop soft centers if steamed. Japanese red or white ginseng is generally regarded as inferior to Chinese or Korean. It is not possible to compare the quality of American and Asian ginseng because their medicinal properties differ. Wild American ginseng is much more expensive in both East and West than any of the cultivated roots. Care should be taken when purchasing ginseng to ascertain its origin.

High cost has also encouraged fraudulent substitutions of other roots for ginseng: for example, *Campanunoea pilosule*, also called "Bastard Ginseng" (tang shen) in China, and *Adenophora verticillata* (shashen). In America, red dock root has sometimes been sold as red ginseng. The Chinese relate a traditional method of telling the real from the fake. Two people are chosen and made to walk four Li (a Chinese mile). One has a piece of the supposed ginseng in his mouth. If at the end of the walk the person with the root does not feel in the least bit tired but the other person is somewhat out of breath, then the drug is true.

THE HISTORY OF GINSENG IN NORTH AMERICA

The American *Panax quinquefolium*, though not trumpeted as a panacea or elixir of life, was still a most useful folk remedy. Shamanistic Indian tribes in the mountains of mid-America used it with more ritual, sorcery, and spirit guidance than the scientifically minded Chinese Taoist herbalists of the time. In the American colonial period, ginseng was wildly advertised by the notorious quack doctors of the white settlements, but so was just about everything else. The official United States Pharmacopeia during the last century listed ginseng as a stomach remedy and stimulant.

North American ginseng cultivation provides an extraordinary economic and social story. It is not commonly known that ginseng digging was the main source of support for some of the early American settlers. The enterprise began in 1716 in Canada, where a Jesuit missionary, Father Lafiteau, discovered a plant similar to the one described by Father Jartoux in China. Avid collection soon began for dispatch to China, which was an unlimited market for

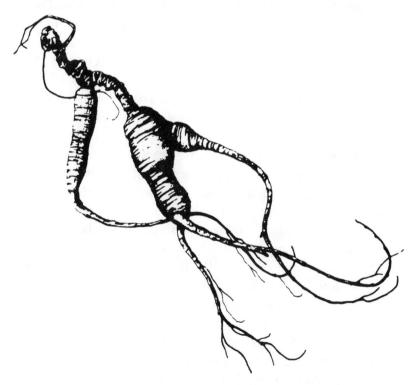

A 41-year-old wild American ginseng root.

ginseng, and boatloads were exported to Canton at a profit so huge that ginseng became second only to the fur trade in profitability.

Indiscriminate picking and inadequate preparation of the roots dried up the Canadian trade by 1760. The United States took over and trade expanded. In 1862, a good year, 622,761 pounds of dried roots were shipped to Canton and Hong Kong. Fur trappers used to return from the mountains with fur and ginseng, and in fact ginseng trade in America today is still carried out by fur companies. Entire villages in Kentucky and Wisconsin used to go out into the forest and, with "mattock and sack," dig for "seng," as it was known. Sometimes they managed to collect bushels of roots in a day. The price rose and rose. A book on Daniel Boone records that he personally collected large amounts of ginseng and purchased more from the white settlers. In the winter of 1787 to 1788, he started up the Ohio in a boat containing nearly fifteen "caggs" (tons) of ginseng, all of which he lost when the boat overturned. Undismayed, by the following autumn he had collected another fifteen caggs.

When wild ginseng became scarce at the end of the nineteenth century, some enterprising farmers attempted cultivation, and a few had great success. However, as already noted, ginseng is liked by other species besides humans and glow-worms; namely, all kinds of insects, fungi, pests, and worms. Virtually the entire American crop was wiped out in 1910, and the Depression finished off many farms. Despite this, cultivation continued in North America, and is now a flourishing industry worth some $50 million a year. Most of this cultivation is concentrated in Marathon County, Wisconsin, with additional crops growing in Ontario, Canada, and throughout the Appalachian Mountains. The majority of this ginseng is exported to the Far East.

There is no reason why ginseng should not be grown in other places that have the cold winters the roots need for winter dormancy, yet there is no report of anyone having done so. Father Lafiteau sent fresh samples from Canada to France, where they were transplanted without success. Ginseng is grown successfully in research centers and state farms in Bulgaria and the Ukraine. The author has supervised a successful five-year agricultural experiment in which ginseng was grown in shade houses on the Golan Heights in Israel. However, the Royal Botanical Gardens in Kew, England, for example, have not even made an attempt. Here is a golden opportunity for someone with a green thumb!

SEARCHING FOR A SUBSTITUTE

The Institute of Biologically Active Substances in Vladivostok, attempting to find substitutes for ginseng because of its rarity and its reluctance to be cultivated, searched through the Araliaceae family and discovered a range of stimulatory and adjustive remedies. The most effective and safest was a thorny shrub called *Eleutherococcus senticosus*, which grows in Siberia, China, and Korea and has medicinal properties similar to those of ginseng. Tests showed that the roots and leaves possess a broad range of tonic effects. Eleutherococcus is now widely used in the former USSR, and is officially recognized as a restorative by the health ministry. It is given not only to athletes and cosmonauts, but also to factory workers and those who are highly stressed, convalescent, or debilitated. In Chinese medicine it is called *ciwuja* and is used somewhat like ginseng, though it is not so strong.

Continued interest in Eleutherococcus stems from its wide availability in the wild. Factories in the Far Eastern provinces of the former USSR now extract Eleutherococcus on a large scale and distribute millions of doses every month. It has become known as Siberian ginseng, or Eleuthero, although in fact it is far from ginseng botanically. Nevertheless, it carries some of the true ginseng's reputation at a quarter of the price and is becoming quite popular in the West, especially among athletes and fitness enthusiasts.

THE WORLD MARKET

Ginseng is now a major world crop, valued by the International Trade Centre of the United Nations at over $200 million at harvest. This would put it at around a billion dollars retail after it has been made into products. Ginseng "currently represents one of the largest currency earners among the medicinal plants," comments the International Trade Centre. In the Far East and among Asian communities in the West, ginseng roots are sold as they are, singly or in boxes of about a pound and a half. Price depends on quality, size, age, region of growing, and shape: the more man-like the root the better. Ginseng is processed into tablets, capsules, instant teas, and other products for Western and (increasingly) young Asian consumers. By the time the ginseng is on sale in the shop—say, in capsules—its price may be five to ten times that of the original dried roots.

The commercial potential of ginseng is also changing official attitudes to it. Fifteen years ago, Westerners were completely dismissive of a medicine that all Easterners regarded as their most potent. Indeed this strange fact aroused my curiosity, and in 1971, first tempted me to start research on ginseng. Today the puzzle has been partly resolved, for the public is not so ignorant of ginseng, and experts are prepared at least to tolerate it, though few understand it. It is now one of the few plants left in the Soviet, Japanese, and Asian pharmacopeias. Significantly, it has recently entered the Swiss, German, and French pharmacopeias, the only new plant to do so for many years. Eventually it will probably be entered in other Western manuals of medicines as well. Ginseng has been so visible in pharmacies for so many years that the authorities cannot help putting it in the official drug lists, if only to help pharmacists distinguish the real thing from its substitutes. Many governments now permit manufacturers of ginseng products to claim on the labels of the packets and in the accompanying literature that ginseng can help relieve tiredness, weakness, and debility. For example, the German health ministry's "Kommission E" defined ginseng's uses: "As a tonic for invigoration and fortification in times of fatigue and debility or declining capacity for work and concentration, and also in convalescence." Thus it would be correct to state that ginseng is truly here to stay.

CHAPTER 4

Beyond Stimulants and Sedatives

Some of the confusion about what ginseng actually does for people—does it pep them up or calm them down?—arises from several sources: the earlier scarcity of scientific evidence, lack of information about the chemical composition of the root and the actions of its various components, and disappointing results among people taking the root in the wrong way or for the wrong reason.

When carefully reviewed, research shows that ginseng is far more than just a simple stimulant or sedative. Complex in its effects, this ancient root appears to actually normalize the body by aiding a variety of functions.

GINSENG AS A STIMULANT

Chinese herbal guides and Chinese medical tradition only briefly mention ginseng as a stimulant that overcomes exhaustion. They concentrate rather on its long-term use for restoration of health and vitality. Such subtle lasting effects on health are difficult to measure with the techniques of modern science, so research has concentrated more on short-term actions. This has emphasized the stimulant effect of ginseng in the eyes of Westerners, but it must be remembered that the emphasis in traditional and herbal medicine is just the reverse.

Ginseng's effectiveness as a short-term stimulant is of great potential interest to Westerners, who are badly in need of a stimulant that does no harm. Ginseng, in fact, is a stimulant that may actually be good for you, depending on your state of health and functioning.

Reviewing the Studies

Some of the earliest experiments on this stimulant action were carried out on mice by Professor Israel I. Brekhman, head of the Institute of Biologically Active Substances in Vladivostok, who devised a test to determine whether ginseng could increase stamina. Mice are put in water, where they swim until they are exhausted. They are allowed to rest and then made to swim a second time. Professor Brekhman showed that mice given ginseng were able to swim nearly twice as long before they were exhausted than when no ginseng was given.

The same experiment has been repeated in many parts of the world, with the same result. A European laboratory has recently demonstrated that even if the mice are given only moderate doses of ginseng—the equivalent to a mouse of what a human might take just for general health maintenance—their increase in stamina is still quite noticeable. The effect is cumulative. If mice are given ginseng continuously for a month, then for two to three weeks afterwards they can swim for twice as long as mice not given ginseng.

The importance of these mice marathons is that they show objectively that ginseng does have marked effects, and that its effects are not merely psychological. The mice are not swimming longer because someone has told them how the Chinese Emperors enjoyed their ginseng or because they saw a ginseng advertisement in the newspaper. The studies also indicate that ginseng can be strong, especially in extreme situations. But they do not tell us much about *how* ginseng works. Similar stamina tests have shown that caffeine, concentrated extracts of certain other plants such as basil, and even conventional anti-depressant drugs increases the energy of mice. Furthermore, the tests are not especially accurate, nor are they particularly humane.

Studies on people can give us more direct information, although they are scientifically less objective. The ginseng plant's effects were first discovered by the sensitive self-observation of herbalist sages typified by the Emperor Shen Nung. Elaboration and understanding of how and when to take it for best results has come to us through millennia of careful observation. Science carries this a stage further. As an engineer assesses the strength of a structure by testing it under an excessive load, so human studies attempt to reveal the effects of ginseng by testing at extremes of stress or exhaustion.

Russian scientists have examined ginseng's effect on human work capacity and energy by giving ginseng to proofreaders, who were then required to concentrate for longer periods than they were used to. Speed and accuracy tests showed that those given ginseng increased the number of letters read by 12 percent and decreased their mistakes by 51 percent compared with those given a "mock extract" without ginseng. Similar results have been obtained when ginseng has been tested among people carrying out other demanding activities, such as high-speed radio telegraphy. It has been shown to improve the performance and capacity of students taking exams at a Swedish university and people doing exhausting physical work. In fact, the first study to convince Soviet scientists that there was something to ginseng, thus leading to verification in laboratories around the world, involved 100 Soviet soldiers on a cross-country run. Those taking ginseng lopped some 6 percent from their times, compared with others taking a similar preparation without ginseng.

I have carried out a study, along with other doctors at the Maudsley Hospital in London, that tests ginseng under a very special condition of stress and tiredness: that of the switch-over from day to night work. Nurses were given either Korean ginseng or a look-alike inert tablet for the first three days of their switch. After the third night, which is the one that they usually feel the most, they were tested for performance, energy, tiredness, ability to sleep during the day, and other indicators of adaptation. As expected, after switching to night work the nurses showed a considerable drop in alertness, energy, proficiency, activity, and ability to work, and they felt below par. Ginseng restored performance and mood more than the inert look-alike: not all the way back to what it was during normal daytime working, but about half way. Although the nurses didn't sleep as well during the day, presumably because of the stimulation of the ginseng, they coped much better at night. This was after only three days at a small daily dose of just about one gram of good quality Korean ginseng, equivalent to that recommended on the labels of most ginseng products in stores.

Contradictory Results?

While the results of much of the research on ginseng as a stimulant have been impressive, all told, study results have been inconclusive. Sometimes it works and sometimes it doesn't. When ginseng has been tested with young and fit people, especially sportsmen, the result has not been very impressive. Studies carried out by Dr. Imre Forgo, Chairman of the Doping Commission of the International Amateur Boxing Association in Basle, Switzerland, showed that ginseng seemed to improve respiration and oxygen levels in the blood during exercise. But other researchers have failed to confirm such effects. A study of fit young marathon runners was carried out at the U.S. Army Research Institute of Environmental Medicine in Natick, Massachusetts. Some took ginseng for four weeks and others a dummy pill. At the end of the period, those taking ginseng showed no advantage in stamina and body function during intensive exercise.

On the other hand, whenever ginseng has been tried with unfit, tired, run-down and older subjects, the results are much more impressive; it always has a quite noticeable effect. For example, a study of 50 patients who were suffering from "burnout" (depression and chronic fatigue) at the University of Buenos Aires, Argentina, showed that after they had taken ginseng for a period of time, all their mind-body functions improved markedly. They were more energetic and alert and less depressed; had better reactions, nervous function, concentration, memory, mood, and motivation; and were more sociable. In a study at the University of Göteberg, Sweden, Dr. Ingela Wiklund and her colleagues tested 480 older volunteers who took either a ginseng-vitamin mixture or a dummy pill. In this case they found that those taking the ginseng were considerably more alert yet relaxed. They performed better in tests of quality of life, which examined mood, sense of being in control, fatigue, level of depression and anxiety, and general well-being.

The studies seem to show that when young and fit

people take ginseng, there is little obvious change in performance, but that when older people who are not in as good a condition take ginseng, the effects are much more noticeable and consistent. The explanation for this can be found within Oriental medicine. As we have seen, it is a clear principle of Oriental medicine that ginseng should have more powerful tonic effects in those that need it—those whose energy is flagging from stress, aging, or any other reason.

A Balanced Remedy

Ginseng stimulates the nervous system. Reflexes have been shown to speed up; for example, tests have shown that the eyes take less time to adjust to the dark after a person takes ginseng. Professor Wesselin Petkov, of the Institute of Advanced Medical Training in Sofia, has been occupied for the last fifteen years with elaborate experiments to assess its effects on the nervous system. He finds a typical pattern of brain wave stimulation on the electroencephalogram when experimental animals are given ginseng, and he has repeatedly observed increases in the speed of conditioned (learned) behavior in both animals and human subjects, which implies an increase in efficiency of cerebral activity.

Professor Petkov has also shown a surprising phenomenon in mice that had learned a certain repetitive behavior pattern. Once they were allowed to forget their training, they could remember it after a single low dose of ginseng (corresponding to less than a gram for a human). Rats given ginseng also showed increased mental adaptability, more easily switching from one type of learned response to another. He concluded from these types of experiments that: "Ginseng stimulates the basic neural processes which constitute the functioning of the cerebral cortex," namely, the excitation and inhibition that form "the physiological basis of man's mental functioning as a whole." In contrast to other stimulants, he continued, "ginseng causes no disturbance in the equilibrium of the cerebral processes. This explains the absence of any pronounced state of subjective excitement as is characteristic of all other stimulants . . . and also why this stimulant does not interfere with the normal course of sleep." He felt that he had discovered a properly balanced stimulant that actually improved the overall function of the mind and brain at no cost in jittery over-arousal or subsequent exhaustion.

To these scientists, ginseng seemed to herald an entirely new generation of substances that in some unknown way could help people to cope more easily with their burdens. "After various kinds of experiments on men," writes Professor Petkov, "it was established that daily doses of ginseng preparations during 15 to 45 days increase physical endurance and mental capacity for work, as well as industrial activity." The increase in work efficiency was noted not only during the treatment itself but also for a month and a half after the treatment was over.

To study how ginseng stimulates, Japanese researchers have simply watched and measured the activity of animals given ginseng extract, compared with others given a similar but dummy liquid. Animals given ginseng showed more general activity. They explored their environment—running up nets and through holes—more frequently than their colleagues. The difference was especially pronounced when the animals were tired from previous exercise.

In keeping with its action on the nervous system, ginseng has been shown to reverse and block the effects of alcohol and such sedative drugs as barbiturates and chlorpromazine. Yet, strangely, it has been demonstrated that there is a sedative component in the root itself. Japanese scientists at the University of Tokyo showed that rats given very high doses of ginseng extract in addition to a sleep medication slept more and were less restless than with the sleep medication alone.

Solving the Paradox

How is it possible for a remedy to have both stimulating and sedative effects? It is indeed possible—and without paradox. It has been shown that ginseng, like most medicinal plants, contains a number of components, some of which can work in opposite ways. Japanese scientists in particular have carried out extensive and highly sophisticated tests of behavior and activity in animals. They find that certain components increase activity and learning ability and others decrease it. The whole root is therefore a combination of both. This is one plausible explanation for the balanced action noticed by Petkov—that alertness is increased but the ability to rest, relax, and sleep is nevertheless preserved.

A remedy that can have apparently opposite effects is no mystery in the herbal tradition. Indeed, such remedies are treasured: The value of a single preparation that can pick you up if you are over-tired yet prevent you from becoming over-excited is obvious.

Ginseng vs. Other Stimulants

As Professors Petkov and Brekhman have remarked, there is a world of difference between ginseng and other stimulants such as caffeine or amphetamines:

- Ginseng is not an excitant. It does not cause feelings of

over-excitation, emotional disturbance, or agitation in humans, nor, as far as can be judged, in animals.

- Ginseng may assist in combating stress, while other stimulants actually can cause stress.

- There is a sedative component in ginseng. Unlike other stimulants, it produces no sleep difficulties.

- Ginseng is most active when most needed. The more tired one is, the more it stimulates.

- Ginseng causes an increase in health, appetite, and mental condition, especially if taken over time. Other stimulants cause more ill health the longer they are taken.

- Ginseng is much safer than other stimulants.

GINSENG AND STRESS

The body has automatic mechanisms that are called upon if a dangerous or potentially harmful situation arises. Loud noises, threats, wounding, potential attack, fear, anger, emotional tension, and other stressors all generate an automatic response, which is controlled by nerves and hormones. The latter are chemical substances, made in various glands, that regulate and integrate metabolism and coordinate the body's response to the world. Like nerves, they send messages, but more slowly; if nerves are the body's telephone system, then hormones are its postal service. Hormones secreted from the adrenal glands, just above the kidneys, govern the stress response, and produce a state of readiness and mobilization. Blood is shifted away from "peacetime" functions, such as digestion, to the muscles. The heart speeds up, blood vessels contract, blood pressure rises, the metabolism changes, the pattern of the body defenses against injury and infection alters, and the mind becomes aroused.

Occasional stress is often necessary and can help keep people alert and motivated, but too much stress is undoubtedly bad. Whether from outside, such as that experienced by busy administrators or workers in a noisy factory, or from inside in tense and anxious people, continuous stress is disastrous for health. It lowers resistance to disease, contributes to high blood pressure and cardiovascular problems, has been implicated in cancer, and may be a direct cause of digestive troubles, gastric ulcer, tiredness, insomnia, migraines, and other diseases. The body is drained of vitality when its defenses are overworked.

Reviewing the Studies

In a study that I carried out with other scientists at Chelsea College, University of London, we tested an idea first put forward by Professor Brekhman—that ginseng helps people overcome stress and challenge. We gave ginseng extract to many mice and the usual inactive extract to a similar number. We watched the general behavior of the mice, then put them in a situation of mild stress by placing them on a large white disc under a light. They find this somewhat alarming, since they are accustomed to corners and dark holes.

Mice that had ginseng could hardly be distinguished from the others during normal activity, but as soon as they were placed under stress, their reactions were much more pronounced. They explored, crouched, and went into their alert defensive rituals a great deal more than those not given ginseng. This means that ginseng improved their capacity to respond to stress.

The major success of scientific research on ginseng is

that it has repeatedly shown that ginseng helps the body to cope with stress. In laboratories in Korea, Russia, Bulgaria, America, and England, mice under stress that were given ginseng showed two basic improvements. First, the adrenal glands increased in weight and function with less abnormal behavior and distress; in fact, the mice were better able to "absorb" stress. (One is reminded of the Chinese soldiers who took ginseng with them to the battlefield.) Second, the long-term stress response and its corresponding harmful effects were reduced; the body had increased its resistance. Animals that took ginseng not only coped better with stress but their body activity settled back to normal more quickly. It is now felt that this is a key to ginseng's reputed ability to increase health.

HELPING THE BODY ADAPT

A consideration of the way ginseng can cause resistance to stress leads inevitably to one of the most exciting ideas in pharmacology. Professor Brekhman, as well as scientists in South Korea, carried out several experiments. Mice that were given ginseng were subjected to the depressant action of chloral hydrate, barbiturates, and alcohol; their recovery improved. They were irradiated with X-rays, the most damaging of influences on the body; their resistance doubled. The mice also showed a greater ability to survive after being given a highly toxic collection of poisons and drugs—such as potent anticancer agents—after infection with bacteria and after stress by physical conditions such as heat, cold, and changes in pressure.

Chemical changes in the body were then measured to see how the mice were coping. The surprising fact is that ginseng had no effect on these processes in the absence of stress. In other words, it only acted to return the body to normal if it had gone off course. This has led to the exciting concept of the plant as an adaptogen; that is, a substance that increases the ability of the body to adapt. The idea is unique in Western drug research, and apart from ginseng and its relatives within Oriental medicine, no other drug or medicine is known to have such a normalizing effect. Most scientists who have been studying the action of drugs would probably find it hard to believe that such a thing exists. But the evidence is published in the scientific literature and is plain for everyone to see.

How can ginseng work as an adaptogen? It is difficult to know exactly, because it has so many different effects on the body. The secret is likely to be in the way that it acts on the hormones. If ginseng improves the efficiency of the hormone messenger systems, then one might expect greater coordination in the body's defense forces. The body is helped to help itself, whether the problem is abnormal blood pressure or abnormal fatigue.

There is evidence that ginseng does indeed stimulate several glands so as to regulate their hormone production. Korean and Chinese research has shown that ginseng acts directly on the adrenal glands, although other studies showed that resistance is improved even when the adrenal glands are removed. We can suggest that some of the actions of ginseng are through the adrenal glands, while others, as Professor Petkov has shown, may be on the brain itself.

ALERTNESS AND CHALLENGE

There is an interesting connection between the way ginseng improves alertness and well-being, and the way it protects against stress and strain. Common sense tells us that there is a natural linkage between mental wakefulness and the stress response. For example, challenge—things that go bump in the night, or the starting gun of an athletic event—is a considerable stimulant to the brain. Too much challenge—continuous anxiety, executive stress, or long hours on the production line—saps available mental energy, leading to exhaustion and the feeling of being drained. Scientists know that challenge wakes up the mind initially through the production of adrenaline. At the same time, the stress hormones, called corticosteroids, are released by the adrenal glands, travel to the brain, and produce motivation, alertness, and a readiness to act, while also travelling to the muscles and circulation to alert them.

There is evidence that ginseng facilitates this linkage between mind and body. To begin with, the kind of wakefulness produced by ginseng is quite similar to that produced by the corticosteroids. It is an increased alertness, motivation, energy, and even well-being, which is also experienced by patients who have received corticosteroids for medical conditions. Experiments in which tired animals have had to negotiate mazes or tired people have had to solve problems or transmit in Morse code also show that ginseng creates a mental readiness and capacity to meet challenge. It is completely different from the "speediness" produced by other stimulants that act by accelerating mental activity.

Studies carried out by Dr. Deepak Shori and myself at the University of London made it clear that ginseng increased the amount of corticosteroid hormones getting to the brain. After giving animals a measured amount of these hormones, much more was found located in the brain of animals given ginseng than those given a dummy preparation. Dr. Susumu Hiai and other scientists at Toyama University in Japan have gone even further. In a long investigation covering years of work, they have shown that ginseng acts on the regulation systems in the brain, located in the glands called the hypothalamus and pituitary, that actually direct the state of readiness in both body and mind. These glands receive messages from the senses calling for mobilization and then tell the adrenal glands to send out their stress hormones. In other words, improved stamina and alertness equals resistance to stress, and both are achieved by more efficient physiological coordination. Ginseng makes a little hormone go a long way.

These modern descriptions correspond exactly to the claims of the ancient Chinese. Their description of ginseng as an "adjustive" or "kingly" remedy we now know means it helps to adapt to stress, and "yang" we know means alerting, arousing, awakening. Ginseng is not alone in this category. Many other "kingly" Chinese plants make certain body functions more efficient. For example, licorice acts on the water balance in the body through other hormones; pantocrine, or deer antler, appears to help in the sexual or generative area; Bupleurum improves liver function; *Schizandra chinensis* tunes the carbohydrate metabolism; *Angelica sinensis* (Dong Kwai) treats disturbances in female hormones and restores poor vitality, especially in women. All of these kingly remedies have the interesting property of having little effect when the body and mind are in good condition, well-motivated, well-functioning, vital, and energetic. They tend to act only when the system is thrown out of balance.

"TUNING" BODY AND MIND

The research just discussed demonstrates how ginseng helps to harmonize mind and body. It is as if ginseng tunes our engines to make them work more efficiently; we get better performance with less fuel. Interestingly, "tuning" and "toning" come from the same word. Ginseng conforms to the original meaning of the word "tonic," an agent that adjusts or "tunes" the body and mind to make it function better.

The Chinese, of course, have recognized this property of ginseng for a long time. They have always stated that ginseng adjusts or harmonizes body functions that have gone astray. They are justified in saying, "I told you so." A harmless medicine that returns wayward body processes to normal, however mild the effect, may be described as an ideal medicine. The medicine of the past may well turn out to be a medicine of the future.

CHAPTER 5

The Active Ingredients

A plant with such subtle properties as those of ginseng irresistibly makes people wonder how it works and what components are responsible for its remarkable actions. Over the years, chemists have tried to take it to bits to analyze its components, but until the early 1960s, the only substances detected in the root were the usual carbohydrates, cellulose, minerals, and other common constituents that you would expect to find in parsnips or potatoes. After that, however, when it had been demonstrated clearly that ginseng could increase the stamina of mice, scientists began to take the root apart chemically and see which agents could achieve the same results as the whole root. The results of these studies raised as many questions as they did answers.

DISCOVERING THE PRINCIPAL COMPONENTS

In the early 1960s, Professor A.B. Elyakov's team at Moscow University and Professor Shoji Shibata's team in Tokyo began a race to find the key ingredients of ginseng, producing a flurry of reports that mystified the rest of the scientific world, which at the time couldn't understand what the fuss was about.

Using modern analytical techniques, they found that compounds called terpenoidal glycosides could give mice as much extra stamina as the whole root. These are somewhat soapy (or oily) materials made up of sugar molecules connected to a terpenoid molecule, a plant hormone whose structure is quite like that of the human corticosteroid hormones we have discussed. The terpenoidal glycosides are distant cousins to such well-known medicinal glycosides as digitalis. Ginseng glycosides are made in the leaves, flowers, and peel of the root and are then transported to the flesh of the root where they are stored. Two to six percent of the dry root may consist of these materials. Twenty different glycosides have now been identified, and their chemical structure revealed. Named *ginsenosides* by Japanese researchers, these substances have been coded Ra, Rb, Rc, and so on. Different ginsenosides vary in proportion according to the way the root is grown, where it comes from, its age, variety, method of drying, and so on. Just before harvest in August, the ginsenosides reach a peak, which becomes higher each year as the plant gets older. There are quite extensive differences between ginseng species: American ginseng can be distinguished from Asian ginseng by having more ginsenosides of less variety, with Ra, Rf, and Rh absent.

Now that the main active materials are known, it is possible to set a standard minimum amount of ginsenosides (usually one or two percent) a product must have for it to be described as pure ginseng. Such a standard was introduced in the 1987 Swiss Pharmacopeia.

Many of the medicinal properties of ginseng root demonstrated in the laboratory can be reproduced with ginsenosides alone. They have been shown to stimulate, reduce stress, affect the adrenal glands and hormones, increase metabolism in the liver and other organs, affect the circulation, and increase stamina, wakefulness, and performance. Some interesting discoveries have emerged; for example, that Re and Rg are more stimulatory, and Rc and Rb are more sedative. Differences in the amounts of each type could explain how some roots—for example, American ginseng—are more yin or quieting, while others—for example, Korean red ginseng—are more yang or arousing.

However, the situation is not yet clear. In some good quality roots, such as six-year-old red ginseng, there will be less ginsenoside than in poor quality ginseng, such as four-year-old pencil roots. Furthermore, even though root hairs and tendrils are of poor quality and less effect, their ginsenoside levels are extremely high. In fact, Koreans traditionally throw away a lot of the ginsenosides when they peel roots for steaming. Finally, infected or damaged roots have more ginsenosides than healthy ones. Considering all these facts, it becomes clear that one cannot make the equation "ginsenosides equal medical effects." As a way out of this problem, it has been suggested that it is not the total amount of ginsenosides in the roots that produces the effects, but the relative quantities of various types. This may be true, but is as yet unproven.

OTHER COMPONENTS

It is more likely that other substances unrelated to the ginsenosides contribute to ginseng's effects. A few are becoming known; most are still unidentified. For example, a unique protein material has been found in ginseng that seems to be responsible for helping in the metabolism of sugar and fat. A group of compounds termed *plant phenols*, in particular maltol, have been found to be antioxidants; they can help protect the tissues and possibly reduce some of the damage due to aging. Special sugar compounds termed *polysaccharides*, which can support the body's immunity, have been found in ginseng. We also know that ginseng contains essential oils, fats, ginsenin, phytosterin, resins, mucilaginous compounds, vitamins, sugars, certain alkaloids, minerals, silicic acids, and other substances. Clearly there are many ingredients in ginseng that add up to its total effect. Ginseng is a good example of an herb in which the whole is greater than the sum of its parts.

IS GINSENG UNIQUE?

A question that might be raised is whether the ginsenosides, or terpenoidal glycosides in general, appear in other plants, and if so, whether they have ginseng-like properties. The ginsenosides are unique and are found only in ginseng and its relatives, but there are other terpenoidal glycosides in many plants, especially those with medicinal properties recognized by Chinese medicine. The kingly remedies have them, as do licorice, jujube, Bupleurum species, Platycodon species, Polygala species (such as snakeroot), and Schizandra. In Western medicine the sedative valerian and the tonics sarsaparilla and spikenard are among the well-known plants in which triterpenoid glycosides—which always have mild, tonic, adjustive effects—could be the active ingredients. It is this mildness that has prevented Western scientists from taking the triterpenoid glycosides seriously. You won't find them in textbooks of pharmacology, because conventional research into drugs is looking for strong curative chemicals, not mild, adjustive, or preventive ones.

CHAPTER 6

Ginseng and Disease

Ginseng does not cure any specific disease or relieve any specific symptom. It can improve general health, vitality, adaptability, or resistance, and thus may prevent or curb a disease. In particular, ginseng may aid in a number of diseases endemic to the modern world as a result of too much stress and strain.

Some 10 percent of Americans suffer from high blood pressure or other circulatory problems known to be strongly influenced by anxiety and tension. In humans, cancer risk is increased by grief or despair, and in laboratory animals, by stress or crowding. Even infections are more readily caught by people in difficult circumstances. The way stress creates holes in our immunity is becoming much clearer today, giving rise to a science with its own name: psychoneuroimmunology. The hormones we have been discussing in regard to ginseng are very much involved in the weakening of immunity by unremitting stress.

Ginseng tightens up the physiological systems that react to stress and so might be expected to reduce the damage created when stress becomes excessive. Thus it should improve resistance to infections—and possibly even cancer—and curtail circulatory and other diseases that arise from inner imbalance. We will examine each of these in turn.

BOOSTING OVERALL IMMUNITY

From 1975 to 1980, no fewer than 60,000 Soviet workers at the Volzhsky car factory in Togliatti were given extract of Eleutherococcus daily for several months. Their general health improved, the number of days off work was substantially reduced, and they seemed to be in better cardiovascular condition than the rest of the workers. Such studies have been carried out with several kinds of Soviet workers, especially long distance truck drivers, although with ginseng relatives rather than ginseng. The Russians have stated that their aim is to reduce ill health among workers made vulnerable by industrial stress. They appear to have succeeded, and both ginseng and Eleutherococcus are now available in the former USSR for this purpose. Similar observations have been reported from Europe, where residents of old people's homes who were given ginseng appear to be rather more healthy, active, and resistant to disease than others. However, it is difficult to prove that it was the ginseng—or other salutary influences—that benefited the patients. The same criticism can be leveled at the Soviet trials, however massive.

Nevertheless there is some scientific support for the claim that doses of ginseng at the right time can help restore weakened resistance. Animals given ginseng and then infected with disease-causing bacteria are less likely to become ill than others. In Japan, researchers have found that ginseng can boost the immune system—both the white cells that stand guard and the antibodies that are their weapons. Ginseng is known to enrich the blood with protective cells, and their manufacture in the bone marrow noticeably speeds up. Studies at the Central Drug Research Laboratory in Lucknow, India, suggest that members of the ginseng family may even be able to stimulate the body to produce more interferon, the antiviral protective protein.

Recent research at the Department of Pharmacology of the University of Milan has found that healthy people, after taking ginseng for eight weeks, had a more powerful immune system that was capable of resisting bacteria, cancer cells, and other unwanted guests in the body compared with those who took dummy pills. Ginseng is not the only remedy that can generally strengthen the immune system. It and certain other herbal remedies, such as Dong Kwai, together with food components such as zinc and vitamin C, are all termed *immunomodulators* because of their support of our resistance.

It is important not to regard ginseng as some kind of antibiotic. It has no effect whatever against bacteria, viruses, or any other infectious agent. Instead it helps shore up immunity that is reduced by exhaustion, strain, or poor vitality. Even in this role ginseng does not provide a quick fix. There are, in fact, many other Asian plants with stronger and more specific effects on immunity. Ginseng should be seen as part of a health maintenance program in the Chinese fashion, in which it works alongside dietary control and a healthy life style.

The situation is similar with regard to convalescence, a period of debility and reduced vitality in which ginseng can be very useful. Again, its role is not to cure disease but to help the body recover its strength after it has won the battle against the disease. This has been investigated in the case of tuberculosis by Soviet and Korean scientists, who find that ginseng and Eleutherococcus have no effect in the acute phase but do shorten the recovery stage. A study of 120 patients in a Korean hospital has demonstrated clearly that ginseng glycosides can aid recovery and shorten the hospital stay of patients who have had serious operations.

CANCER

Insofar as cancer arises through depressed immunity, ginseng may have a general preventive effect against it, especially when combined with healthy habits. The restoration of vitality and well-being makes cancer less likely. Ginseng has no effect on cancer itself, just as it has none on invading bacteria. The one important potential use of ginseng in cancer is for support during treatment, which is stressful, debilitating, and damaging to immunity. Although treatment can destroy primary cancers, the patient is often left more vulnerable to secondaries. Animal studies by Dr. K.V. Yaremenko and his colleagues in the former USSR have indicated that Eleutherococcus can protect the body from the stress of surgery and chemotherapy and prevent the increased risk of secondary growths. Korean scientists have reported similar findings with ginseng. Both Eleutherococcus and ginseng also have been shown to protect patients from some of the damage and debility caused by radiotherapy. Patients are better able to tolerate treatment and have fewer side effects such as nausea and tiredness. At the famous Petrov Oncological Institute in Leningrad, one teaspoon of concentrated Eleutherococcus extract daily enabled patients to cope successfully with 50 percent higher doses of anticancer drugs, with resulting longer life.

Ginseng and especially Eleutherococcus are now used quite widely for this purpose in the former USSR. A range of specialized plant remedies are also used in China to assist the health and immunity of patients during medical treatment of cancer. (This subject is discussed further in my recent book *How to Survive Medical Treatment*.) That they have been doing this for 20 years without Western doctors taking any notice indicates, unfortunately, that conventional medicine is still concentrating on assaulting the disease, leaving the patient unprotected on the battle-field.

CIRCULATORY DISORDERS

Studies have also shown that ginseng may be useful in the all-too-common diseases of the circulation. Ginseng somewhat lowered artificially raised blood pressure in dogs and produced a consistent but small reduction in blood pressure among elderly patients. However, it significantly normalized sharply reduced blood pressure in animals. Ginseng, being a yang or heating remedy, tends to raise (or "heat up") low blood pressure more quickly and easily than it lowers high blood pressure. After a number of clinical studies in Chinese hospitals, the Chinese now use ginseng as part of emergency treatment to restore blood pressure and stabilize patients after shock—for example, from loss of blood—or heart attacks. It appears to be more effective than any conventional drug used for this purpose, especially when combined with other herbs. At the same time, Soviet and German doctors report that ginseng does help to reduce high blood pressure but only as part of a global nature-cure treatment that includes diet or fasting, exercise, and relaxation. In this situation, ginseng would help the body adjust to its new life style, burn up waste products, and stabilize metabolism. Several studies suggest that ginseng reduces cholesterol in the circulation. This is not a primary action—it is not a specific cholesterol-lowering agent—but is secondary to readjustment to a more active, cleaner metabolism. Interestingly, because American ginseng is more yin and less arousing, it may be more successful in this regard than Asian ginseng. According to Dr. Charles Elson at the University of Wisconsin, American ginseng is quite successful at lowering cholesterol levels in laboratory animals.

How ginseng can both lower and raise blood pressure may seem puzzling, but the puzzle is not created by ginseng. It arises from Western assumptions that a drug ought to change some body process in one direction only. In Eastern medicine, remedies that work in more than one direction are the norm. The action of adjustive or adaptogenic medicines depends on the background. They help the body to adapt to its environment by acting as required, raising, lowering, or doing nothing according to the patient's needs.

DISORDERS OF METABOLISM

Diabetes is a disturbance of the metabolism of sugar that is related to impaired insulin activity. Administration of ginseng tends to reduce blood sugar in animals in which it has been artificially raised. This stabilizing effect is typically adaptogenic, since ginseng also raises blood sugar that has been artificially lowered (by insulin injections). It can help to stabilize blood sugar levels but does not replace medical treatment such as insulin for people with diabetes or disorders of sugar metabolism. In China, ginseng and other herbs may be given to people with diabetes as a way of helping their bodies adjust to insulin treatment. Acupuncture plays a similar role in Chinese medicine. It may be more helpful than ginseng alone for allaying some of the potential damage to the tissues that occurs even when the diabetes is treated with insulin.

Ginseng has a subtle effect on many types of metabolism, and research is now being conducted to try to understand its action on chemical processes in the body. Dr. E.V. Aviakian and colleagues at the University of California have recently discovered, for example, that it achieves more economical use of body energy during exercise and extra storage of energy-producing compounds in the liver. The scientists found that if animals are forced to perform extensive exercise, ginseng prevents depletion of the energy supply and reduces the build-up of lactic acid waste products, which cause tiredness. Ginseng can also raise the basal metabolic rate when it is too slow, thus increasing the breakdown and metabolism of foods, liberating more energy, and removing more waste products. (These metabolic effects may be responsible for the suggestion that ginseng can prevent hangovers. Certainly the Russians think it can; they encourage people to take Eleutherococcus or ginseng with or after vodka, and an Eleutherococcus vodka is for sale in Russia.) Ginseng also increases the rate of manufacture of important body chemicals in the liver. It is not certain if these are direct effects of ginseng or secondary results of the stimulation of the hormone system. Interestingly, ginseng can stimulate the metabolism of body cells even when the cells are isolated and kept in a test tube, so hormones are not always required for it to work.

LACK OF SEXUAL VITALITY

One of the many fabled powers of ginseng is the ability to

increase sexual vitality. Science says that ginseng cannot stimulate sexual performance, except in a psychological or suggestive manner. If someone believes that ginseng increases sexual prowess, then it probably will, because virility is to some extent a matter of confidence.

Many herbs and drugs have hopefully been called aphrodisiacs, but there are in fact very few real aphrodisiacs, and it is doubtful if ginseng is one. On the other hand, there is scientific evidence that it may have the less dramatic but nevertheless important function of helping to reverse male impotence when it is not psychological, but is due to a decline in the hormones that control the sexual responses. There is clear evidence that ginseng contains compounds with sex hormone activity, and in some experiments it has been shown to reverse harmful effects caused by lack of male sex hormones.

In other experiments, ginseng glycosides were able to encourage development of sex organs in young animals. Young mice given ginseng reached puberty faster than untreated mice, and their prostate glands were 40 to 60 percent larger. In fact, Professor Brekhman has suggested that the increase in weight of these glands could be used to measure the strength of different ginseng preparations. Dr. K. Karzel of the University of Bonn concludes: "The occurrence of constituents with sex-hormone-like activity in ginseng preparations thus seems to be proven . . . but questions concerning the ratios between male and female hormones remain to be solved."

There are clinical reports from Russia of striking improvements when ginseng was given to some patients suffering from sexual impotence. They felt more tranquil and active and showed an improvement in sexual function. Although much more study is needed, we can say that perhaps the Chinese are justified in expecting to be sexually active in old age with the help of ginseng.

Swallowing the Ginseng Pill

In this chapter, you might say that I've quite literally tried to convince you to swallow a bitter pill—in this case, an herbal one. On the surface, prescribing an herb for diseases that it will not cure seems to ring of pure quackery. But when we seriously consider what we know of ginseng, culling our information from sources ranging from the oldest traditions to the most up-to-date scientific studies, we come to understand the many health benefits of this most often misunderstood and dismissed root.

Clearly, ginseng is no antibiotic. Yet we know that it boosts immunity. It will not cure cancer. But it will support the health and immunity of patients undergoing medical treatment for cancer. It is not a specific cholesterol-lowering agent. But, when combined with other herbs and a global nature-cure treatment, it has been found to aid the maintenance of a clean and active metabolism. And although it is doubtful whether ginseng is an aphrodisiac, it has been shown to contain compounds with sex-hormone activity.

The bottom line, as suggested by the available evidence, is that ginseng works in real yet *subtle* ways to assist the body in combatting disease and maintaining optimum health.

CHAPTER 7

Ginseng and Aging

O f all the people who treasure ginseng in China, the old are most enthusiastic. As we have seen, the common belief is that if taken regularly, it will retard the aging process, keep crippling disorders such as arthritis and cardiovascular disease at bay, provide energy to old people with flagging vitality, and even allow men to retain sexual potency until the very last years of life. The very best gift an old man or woman could receive in China would be a good ginseng root.

Much of the lore and ritual concerning the use of ginseng is perpetuated by the elderly. They are the ones who keep ginseng soaking in brandy for years while they wait for the most auspicious occasion to consume it, who respect ginseng for its supposed radiation and keep it in lead-lined boxes, and who may spend their life's savings on select roots.

Can ginseng really help a man resist the effects of aging? This is really two questions. Is such a thing as a Fountain of Youth possible? If so, would ginseng qualify? To answer these questions we have to know something more about aging.

THE AGING PROCESS

Growing old is inevitable. Despite the biblical statement that Methusaleh and others lived many hundreds of years, it is accepted that potential human life expectancy is limited to about 110. Long before this age the body begins to run down. The functioning of the organs, cells, and metabolism slowly deteriorate. Scientists have demonstrated that the very information that controls the construction and smooth running of the body wears out, just as the message on a tape becomes obscured after many re-runs through a tape recorder. This is the aging process. As it continues, the body becomes more and more vulnerable to disease and damage. Old people are increasingly likely to get infections, for example, and tend to have slower reactions, making them more likely to be involved in traffic accidents.

ATTEMPTS TO RESIST THE EFFECTS OF AGING

Suppose it were possible to increase the resistance of the body so that while aging continued at its own pace, no premature illnesses would occur. In that case, people would reach their potential life span and would be healthy and active until the day they just died of old age, when the body could not function any more. In some areas of the world—secluded valleys in the mountains of South Russia, Hunza in Pakistan, Vilcabambas in Ecuador—there are communities in which significant numbers of very old people are healthy and reach their maximum potential life span of 100 years or just over.

In general, any treatment that improves health and fitness can be expected to aid in resisting the effects of aging, even as aging continues. Yoga and exercise can affect life span in this way. Conversely, cigarette smoking can shorten life by making the body more vulnerable to bronchial infections, emphysema, and cancer.

Every culture has traditional remedies and treatments that are purported to result in healthy long life. In the West, a variety of possible substances have been popular, including vitamins C and E, unsaturated oils in food, procaine, other antioxidants (similar to food preservatives), and synthetic hormones. In addition, rosemary, licorice, garlic, and vegetarian food are traditional suggestions.

In India, a special section of traditional medicine, called Rasaaynen, is devoted to resisting the effects of aging. This treatment, which is of great antiquity and complexity, involves an elaborate regimen of herbs taken over a long period while the subject is living inside a specially built room or cell, the precise measurements of which are prescribed. Some noted Indian politicians, such as Jawaharlal Nehru, are known to have undergone this treatment.

In China, Mao Tse-tung and Chou en-Lai were both known to take ginseng regularly. Father Jartoux was also in complete agreement with the Chinese belief that ginseng was able to prolong life and wrote enthusiastically about it. The Chinese, of course, have a rich source of various herbal medicines that are useful in combating the symptoms of aging, but none has the same repute as ginseng. The New York Times report (in 1933) about a Peking professor who lived for 256 years should not be taken too seriously, but it is of interest that he attributed his purported longevity to a tea he brewed daily. It contained ginseng and "Fo ti teng," which is either *Hydrocotyle asiatica,* a common creeping plant, or the Chinese medicine *Polygonum multiflora.*

The Chinese have always been interested in old age. While European alchemists were devoted to the attempt to convert dross into gold, Chinese alchemists were similarly occupied with finding the elixir of life. The herbal manuals are insistent that ginseng can prolong life, although they recognize that it certainly is not the fabled Elixir of Immortality: "If even the herb Chu-seng can make one live longer, try putting the Elixir in the mouth" says an alchemist book of AD 142. But scientists admit that a real elixir of life is not foreseeable. The aging process cannot be altered or manipulated by any external agent. Immortality is a myth and will remain so. However, this is not so gloomy as it sounds, because the effects of aging can indeed be modified. The motto of the American Gerontological Society is "To Add Life to Years, Not Years to Life."

HOW GINSENG HELPS

In the early twenties, the distinguished physiologist Claude Bernard introduced a fashion for eating the gonads of monkeys to prolong life. Scientists at the time believed that aging was due to the failure of hormones, and that taking hormones in this form could slow the process. A rather less crude type of hormone therapy arrived with the availability of synthetic hormones such as testosterone, which is still taken but only in special cases of premature impotence or decline in virility. It has certain harmful side effects with prolonged use. In theory, hormone therapy could slow down some of the effects of aging, because the efficiency of the hormones in the body does indeed decline with age. Taking hormones may compensate, but only for a limited period.

The Chinese find European involvement with monkey glands amusing. Why, they ask, does one need to eat monkey glands when there is a much more effective, longer lasting, and safer natural remedy? The intriguing fact is that ginseng not only seems to act very much like a hormone but also stimulates the body to produce its own hormones. This may be one way in which it could moderate the effects of aging.

There are other ways, too. We have also seen how a decline in resistance to the wear and tear of life is a key manifestation of aging. Ginseng is almost the only substance known to increase bodily resistance to stress. Another complaint of the elderly is tiredness, and we have demonstrated that ginseng is a safe and effective long term stimulant. All these factors would suggest that ginseng is ideal for treatment of the symptoms of aging.

Unfortunately, there is little scientific evidence. It would be difficult to demonstrate an effect on the life expectancy of humans, because that would take so long that the scientists might not be alive at the end of the experiment. Animals can be used, however. Observations on the effect of ginseng on the life span of mice, which is two years, have been carried out by myself and others at the University of London. Mice were given very small doses of ginseng throughout life. Treated mice appeared more active than those not given ginseng. However, the average and maximum life spans remained about the same for treated and untreated mice. We feel the doses used may have been too small. Soviet scientists have reported that a colony of rats given higher doses of ginseng lived considerably longer than a similar colony without, although this awaits confirmation.

It is also possible to carry out experiments on human cells isolated from the body. Ginseng has been shown by myself and other scientists to stimulate the growth of such cells and delay the death and disintegration of cells when they were under stress. Such experiments are just the beginning.

Human Research

Trials of ginseng among old people in hospitals and old-age homes are also getting under way, and have already given encouraging results. In one case, 66 patients age 30 to 60 were given ginseng and vitamins. Improvements were noticed in most of those who suffered from cardio-vascular diseases, depression, and reduced vitality. Many of the patients showed an awakening interest in life. Such psychological benefits are also the most marked feature of a German clinical trial of ginseng among 95 patients in old-age homes. Besides improvements in blood pressure, memory, neurological function, and bodily function, 58 of the patients showed   an enhancement of mood so marked as to be almost euphoric, and in almost all cases it was maintained for a period of months." The doctors continue: "It goes without saying that tiredness or exhaustion were among our patients' main symptoms....83 percent showed clear improvements in both these syndromes, which can be considered an excellent result."

Dr. Mohan Kataria, a consultant gerontologist of St. Francis's hospital in London, with myself and a nurse, Beryl Gethyn-Smith, have recently studied the effects of good quality Korean red ginseng root on 60 old people who complained of being tired and run down. They took three capsules of ginseng daily for ten days, and on another occasion took a look-alike preparation for ten days. The study was "double blind," that is, neither the old people nor the nurse who evaluated them knew which was which. We found that when they took ginseng there was clear improvement in alertness, speed of reaction, and coordination at tasks that we set for them. Although most of them didn't seem to notice any change in themselves and did not report that they felt any better, a few stated they felt more energetic and active.

Still, it may be true to say that ginseng is ideal for old people. It is my belief that the Chinese have introduced to the world the only drug or medicine ever shown to have medicinal powers that specifically fit the conditions of the elderly. Others who have done research on ginseng also hold this view. Professor Brekhman has been claiming for many years that ginseng would be of great interest to gerontologists (those who study aging). One international company has for some time been marketing a geriatric tonic preparation that is available worldwide. Its main constituent is ginseng.

Not an Elixir of Life

A note of caution is necessary, because it can be dangerous to raise false hopes. We have shown that ginseng cannot be regarded as a panacea. It can only palliate the effects of aging, and even this it does in a mild and gentle manner, building up over a long period. Like many other herbs, it works gradually, and the effects are not dramatic. Moreover, it cannot be expected to cure the degenerative diseases of old age. It is likely to produce a mild improvement, but its main function is to help the body resist developing these conditions in the first place. For this purpose it must be taken continuously and regularly. It is well known that people vary considerably in their response to drugs and herbs, and the effects of ginseng may not be immediately noticeable, depending on such other factors as diet and the quality of the root.

It should be obvious, though, that ginseng cannot be a

substitute for proper self-care. Basic methods of keeping fit and healthy will do more to help you attain a good old age than any tonic, including ginseng. Diet should be moderate, with plenty of roughage, fresh fruit, and vegetables or grains, and with less fat, sugar, starch, and animal products, and fewer rich foods. Exercise should be regular, sufficiently vigorous, and maintained throughout life, because it is difficult and even dangerous to begin vigorous exercise in advanced age. Stress-free living—a sanguine and calm existence—and intelligent avoidance of harmful environmental influences are also essential to health at any age.

CHAPTER 8

When and How to Take Ginseng

As you have seen in earlier chapters, ginseng offers a variety of benefits for the healthy person, and offers relief from a number of disorders, as well. This chapter reviews the many applications of this complex root, provides guidelines for choosing the best ginseng roots and products, and explains how ginseng can be used to best effect.

GINSENG APPLICATIONS

Both modern research and long usage in the East have demonstrated that ginseng can enhance health in a number of ways. The following discussions highlight its most common usage.

Use As a Stimulant

Ginseng has been shown to be a safe, effective, and natural stimulant with many advantages over other stimulants such as caffeine or amphetamines. It can be taken for tiredness and exhaustion or when going through heavily taxing tasks, such as examinations, long-distance driving, stage performances, unusually strenuous physical work, and so on. It is ideally suited for exhaustion from overwork, insomnia, or over-indulgence and may be a most effective way of coping with a hangover. In all these cases it should be taken at the time when it is needed—as opposed to sustained use for other purposes.

Use As a Tonic

The Chinese tend to pay less attention to such immediate uses and more to ginseng as a long-term restorative, because they believed that the benefits to health of natural medicines accrue only from gradual and continuous use. It is especially recommended for convalescence from disease, coping with long-term tiredness, or counteracting the feeling of being below par. Taking ginseng at these times may not only remove the feeling of being tired and "off" but also decrease the likelihood of incurring a disease because of lowered resistance. It may also be taken for the tiredness that accompanies diseases such as anemia and dysentery.

Enhance Mental Health

Judging from Russian experience with ginseng for improving the mental state of the elderly, psychological benefits also may be obtained from long-term use. It can be recommended for depression and insomnia, as it has been documented repeatedly that it can raise spirits and improve outlook on life, especially among the elderly. Its general tonic effects may assist memory and concentration.

Counteract Stress

Ginseng taken regularly may assist in coping with the tensions and strains of life. It may also help the body resist the harmful long-term effect of stress which, as we have seen, can produce a general deterioration of health and well-being.

Help Regulate Blood Pressure

Ginseng may have a mild stabilizing effect on either low or high blood pressure. However, blood pressure problems often result from changes inherent in the cardiovascular system, which cannot be reversed or cured by ginseng. It can be taken safely as a regular course by those with disorders of the cardiovascular system but only on a trial and error basis, with the full knowledge and consent of the individual's doctor. Ginseng normally can be taken in addition to any other prescribed drugs.

Help Control Diabetes

As there is some evidence that ginseng can adjust the blood sugar level in diabetes, it may be taken along with other treatment, and if there is a noticeable improvement this can be considered in the long-term management of the disease. Again, there are no problems of incompatibility with other treatments, as the herb is mild and extremely safe.

Treat Impotence

As we have seen, impotence may be psychological more often than physical. Ginseng may help only certain cases of physical impotence, particularly those resulting from general lack of vitality. Chinese doctors have placed great faith in long-term courses of ginseng for the treatment of such cases, especially the decline in potency that accompanies aging. Incidentally, the Chinese say that when it is used for the treatment of flagging vitality (both sexual and otherwise), it should be accompanied by a period of continence. They believe this causes secretions that arise through the use of ginseng to become reabsorbed into the blood stream so they revitalize the brain and body. The herb is not an aphrodisiac in the sense that it is to be taken at the time of sexual activity to increase virility.

Relieve the Effects of Alcohol, Drugs, and Therapies

Ginseng can be used to overcome intoxication or hangover from drink and to relieve lethargy, tiredness, and poor vitality arising from such drugs as sedatives or tranquilizers, or occurring as side effects of strong medical treatment. In particular, it can be used to help retain some vitality and resistance during chemotherapy or radiotherapy.

However, ginseng should be used with care, because it may sometimes mask a symptom that should be attended to. For example, tiredness associated with drug use is sometimes the result of liver damage, which should be treated accordingly.

Resist the Effects of Aging

As described more fully in Chapter 7, for this purpose ginseng must be taken regularly—at least one course a year, increasing in frequency with age, so that after middle age some is taken every day.

GINSENG DOSAGE

The label on a packet of ginseng may state a recommended dose. How reliable are these instructions? How much of the root should one take? Does the dose depend on the intended purpose? Guidance in these matters, too, can come from a synthesis of Chinese traditional usage, with its thousands of years of experience, and the careful analysis of modern science.

The Chinese chew pieces of ginseng varying in size from a pea to a walnut, usually more than one piece a day. This would correspond to a dose of several grams a day, which is recommended in the Chinese pharmacopeias. However, this is at least twice as much as is usually recommended in Western preparations. This may be because the Chinese are more confident about ginseng than are Europeans. Indeed, the amounts taken by the Chinese sometimes seem to be dictated by how much they can afford rather than any other consideration. Moreover, the quality of the Chinese root is sometimes better than the root commonly available in the West, which would make the actual difference in dosage even greater. Herbal books and sources generally prescribe a dosage of approximately two grams (7/100 ounce) of root daily, split into morning and evening doses.

However, dosage is to some extent an individual matter, and everyone should experiment to find the best dose. A course of ginseng should last for at least a month. Older people can take ginseng continuously for a long time. For a short-term effect—for example, as a stimulant to combat fatigue and exhaustion or in cases of weakness during convalescence—the dose may be increased somewhat. In such cases, three grams a day would probably suffice, split into morning and evening doses. But, again, there is a correct amount for each person, depending on factors such as constitution, the reason for taking ginseng, diet, age, and state of health. People should try to find the dose that is right for them by starting low and increasing the dosage until they hit the level at which they notice positive effects.

SELECTING GINSENG

Because there are so many varieties of ginseng grown in different places, so many products on sale, and a good deal of confusion between Oriental *Panax ginseng*, American *Panax quinquefolium*, and Russian *Eleutherococcus senticosus*, people often don't know which type of ginseng they should purchase. Indeed, there are interesting differences in quality and usage between different varieties and species of the root.

Understanding the Three Main Types of Ginseng

Asian ginseng is the classical ginseng about which so much has been written and researched. It is effective in all the ways discussed in this book and is one of the most important of all restorative herbs. It is the ideal stimulating tonic, being generally more effective than other species. It shouldn't be taken by people with especially nervous, hyperactive, or "hot" dispositions, except for exhaustion, convalescence, or aging. It is the ginseng to take if your constitution and metabolism tend to be "cool," which increases the risk of degenerative diseases. This ginseng tends to be masculine, which means it may amplify male hormonal qualities more successfully than other varieties. Thus it will be better for males than females, although this difference is slight and is pertinent only before menopause. In old age, most people need the "heat" or extra energy provided by this species.

American ginseng is currently available in the United States and the Far East, where it is almost as popular among Asians as is the native species. It does not have the same reputation for bringing life to the old and tired, but it is as useful as the Asian species in balancing or harmonizing the metabolism and reducing stress. Moreover it is a yin tonic, quite suitable for people who are already highly active, energetic, nervous, or choleric, and who wish to take ginseng for its adaptogenic activity without further stoking their fires. There is no difference in its male and female qualities, according to traditional sources, and it can be taken by either sex. In the Far East, American ginseng tends to be preferred in hot climates, as it is slightly cooling, whereas Asian ginseng, which is warming, is preferred in cold climates.

Eleutherococcus, sometimes wrongly called Siberian ginseng, is somewhat like a weak Asian ginseng. The Chinese, who call it ciwuja, have experience in directly comparing it with true ginseng; they regard it as a mildly stimulating tonic of special benefit in restoring metabolic energy. It may be as good as ginseng in its adaptogenic effects on blood circulation and metabolism and costs much less. However, it does not have anything like the Asian ginseng's strength as a restorative for increasing vitality and well-being.

Understanding Grades and Varieties

It is essential to know roots if you wish to get the best from ginseng. You cannot expect to obtain the glowing health promised in the Asian tradition by using cheap ginseng tablets. There are many varieties and grades of root, and each growing country has its own grading system. Furthermore, the main growing countries—China, Korea, Japan, and the United States (in the case of American ginseng only)—have different reputations for quality.

Chinese ginseng is the best marketed in the West but is available only with difficulty from Asian practitioners and suppliers. It varies in quality from absolutely supreme, unavailable from any other country, to middle quality. The finest ginseng, called Yi Sun, may cost hundreds of dollars for an ounce. It is wild ginseng transplanted into a forest bed and maintained there for several years or partly wild ginseng grown from cultivated seed in wild conditions. A slightly lower grade is Pa-Huo Tassel ginseng, which is a very old plant left in cultivated fields for many years (some say over 16) after the rest of the roots are harvested. Shiu Chu ginseng is cultivated in the best possible way and is of top quality, priced at perhaps $50 to $100 an ounce. These grades are all white roots, dried and sometimes preserved with sugar. More commonly available is Kirin ginseng, previously known as Imperial ginseng, which is simply good quality whole root of reasonable age and size. Finally there are small roots, pieces, tails, and the like, which go into root powder and extracts arriving in Western markets as capsules, tablets, teas, and other such products. Their quality is discussed later.

Korean ginseng can be excellent, ranging in quality from very good roots, on the level of Chinese Shiu Chu, down to poor material, below the Chinese. Some Korean roots may be derived from cultivated ginseng transplanted into the wild, as in top Chinese grades, but these do not appear to reach the West. The top Korean grades are all red ginseng, classified as Heaven grade, Earth grade, and Man grade. Because the government controls quality, the Koreans have managed to produce a large amount of excellent ginseng. Poorer quality imitations issue from Hong Kong, so the buyer should check that a Korean red ginseng tin bears the seal of the Office of Monopoly in Seoul. Heaven grade red ginseng roots may cost up to $50 an ounce, depending on the size of the roots. Their advantage is that their quality is guaranteed and they are widely available all over the world. Korea also produces white ginseng of middle quality, as well as Kiboshi, the usual tails, pieces, and pencil roots used to make extracts and products. John Teeguarden, an American who has made a long practical study of the subject, writes in his book, *Chinese Tonic Herbs*, that Korean ginseng is "quicker in its action and is generally more blatant" than the Chinese. "It tones up the Yang as well as the Yin, so it will increase the fire energy, thus stimulating sexual drive and assertive, willful behavior. It is therefore not recommended for people with Yang, hot conditions, but is excellent for those who lack Yang energy." Chinese ginseng is a little less yang, and therefore may be better for long-term restorative use.

Japanese ginseng is middle to poor in quality. Some roots of very good quality are equivalent to the upper grades of Korean ginseng, but these do not often appear in the Western market. Most Japanese ginseng is poor even though it is steamed to make it red, and it looks as good as Korean red roots. Indeed some Japanese roots may be very large, misleading those who wrongly assume size equals quality. Most of these poor Japanese roots find their way to Hong Kong, where they appear as imitation Korean.

Guidelines for Selecting the Root

Ginseng roots are sold singly or packaged into boxes weighing one catty (a little more than a pound). Within each grade the roots are classified into sizes, described by the number of roots that fit into a catty. Thus Earth grade 15 (15 roots to the catty) is better than Earth grade 20 (20 roots to the catty). Although usually the larger the root, the better, grades are a more reliable indication of medicinal value than size; for example, a small root of Heaven grade is better than a large root of Earth grade.

There are some general indications of quality that are worth knowing about besides grades:

- *Age.* The older the root when harvested, the better, which is probably why larger roots are more desirable within each grade.

- *Color.* Generally, red is better than white because only higher quality roots are selected for steaming to produce the red. However, some white roots—particularly the top grade Chinese—are superior to red, and some red roots are poor.

- *Density.* The root should be very hard. If it is red, it should be glassy or crystalline and deep in color.

- *Taste.* The taste of the ginseng root should be rich, strong, and bitter, with an edge of sweetness. If a root is tasteless, don't buy it.

- *Shape.* A good root is straight with intertwined rootlets or branches, sometimes giving it a man-like appearance. Curled roots are of lower quality.

Guidelines for Selecting
Extracts, Tablets, and Teas

Roots are undoubtedly best, and no ginseng cognoscente would touch processed products of any kind, because they are invariably made from poor quality roots. On the other hand, most people just want an effective, cheap, easy-to-take restorative, whether ginseng or something else. In examining products, it should be kept in mind that none of them reaches the standard of the root, although they are certainly less expensive.

One of the problems is that products are often made by Western companies that do not know a great deal about ginseng but buy ground root powder on the international market, then put it into capsules or tablets. This powder may well be poor material to begin with and sometimes is further diluted with fillers, such as lactose, on its way to the consumer. Various analytical tests have been made on ginseng products and a significant portion of them found to contain little or no detectable ginsenosides. A way around this is to choose a Korean or a Chinese product exported to the West in its original packaging. These are almost invariably of better quality. Another way to ensure that you get what you pay for is to buy "standardized" ginseng extract in tablets or capsules. Standardization is a way of processing the ginseng root that guarantees a proper amount of ginsenoside active ingredients (by analysis) in every dose. Of course, it is also advisable to purchase tablets or capsules from the most reputable company.

Thick paste extracts produced in Korea and China can be as good as any product. Ginseng tea should be avoided altogether. You can buy packaged instant teas, made from the root and sometimes the leaf or flower of the plant, which are tasty but medicinally ineffective. In the Far East today one can buy ginseng candies, chewing gum, hair lotion, creams and cosmetics, soup flavorings, and even ginseng cigarettes. Don't expect any tonic effects from these products, either.

TRADITIONAL WAYS OF TAKING GINSENG

The rituals of China concerning the consumption of ginseng are as important as those for cultivation or harvest, even though almost any convenient way of taking it would be medically acceptable. Much of the ginseng in China is boiled and extracted for long periods with water or water and alcohol to give a dark extract, which is sold commercially in a number of closely related forms. Drops of the extract are taken neat or put into tea. A nugget of the required size may be cut from the root and chewed thoroughly until it is completely soft and then swallowed. Another popular method is to make a tea, using special silver kettles because it is a firm rule that no other metal can come into contact with the root. The general tradition is to boil the root for six to ten hours, starting in the evening, then to get up at dawn, drink the preparation, and go back to sleep. It is also common, especially among old people, to put a whole root, together with some leaves if possible, in a bottle of brandy. This is then stored for a long time, after which glasses of it are taken regularly with the greatest relish.

NOTICING THE EFFECTS OF GINSENG

It is a common observation that some people notice the effects of ginseng and others do not. In general, most people notice a stimulation with higher doses, but this depends on whether they are exhausted or not. The more exhausted they are, the more they will notice a return to normal. During the long-term use of ginseng in lower doses, people may not be conscious of any change, because there are enormous constitutional differences in the way people respond. Thin people, for example, tend to be more sensitive to drugs, and someone on a frugal diet may notice the effects of ginseng more than someone who eats meat and rich food.

Ginseng is no more "an alternative to pot and alcohol," as one sensation-seeking news article claims, than is garlic. On the other hand, it can undoubtedly generate a feeling of health and vitality, and therefore a sense of well-being. Some people get the same feeling from a sauna, but it would be an exaggeration to say that saunas make people high. It can be stated categorically that there are no grounds for suggesting ginseng has any intoxicating effect. On the contrary, it has been shown to protect the body from intoxication by alcohol and other drugs. It would thus be more accurate to say that ginseng helps you recover from marihuana and alcohol.

HOW SAFE IS GINSENG?

It has already been mentioned that ginseng is remarkably safe, even in large doses or when taken over a long period. This has been confirmed by modern research. Professor Brekhman writes that a harmful dose for animals has been shown to be at least 1,000 times the effective dose—the equivalent of a man eating three to four pounds of pure ginseng at one sitting. More recently, Professor J. Savel of the pharmaceutical faculty of Paris University tried to give sufficient ginseng to mice to cause side effects. He failed: the mice suffered from enlarged stomachs due to overeating but otherwise remained well.

Italian scientists gave large doses of ginseng to mice continuously for six months without any noticeable ill effects, and clinical trials with patients have never done any harm. Monitoring agencies such as the Food and Drug Administration accept that ginseng is safe and allow it on open sale, without restriction.

It is nevertheless important to realize that after all, ginseng is a medicine, and there are no medicines that don't have some unwanted effects under some conditions. A recent survey by an American doctor showed that some young people who had been taking excessive amounts of ginseng for long periods experienced various symptoms, including insomnia, over-excitation, nausea, and raised blood pressure. One reason for these side effects could be that the young people also took a lot of caffeine and so became over-stimulated. During a trial of ginseng in the Kaschenko Hospital in Russia, "sexual excitement was found to have been produced as a side effect" among some patients taking ginseng for depression. Similar observations, including reports of a temporary return of menstruation after menopause and of breast tenderness in elderly women, have appeared in British medical publications. Whether such effects are harmful enough to outweigh the benefits of ginseng is a decision to be made by the consumer.

Ginseng is safe, but should not be abused. The Chinese tradition states that the young and healthy need no more than an occasional course of ginseng, and only the sick, debilitated, and aged may take it all the time. Over-arousal can sometimes result if excitable and highly strung people take ginseng or if it is taken with other stimulants, such as coffee. For best effects, Asian ginseng should be taken in autumn or winter rather than in the heat of summer.

It is clear that ginseng is not toxic in itself. If taken by the right person at the right time in the right way, its effects will be maximal, and if taken by the wrong person at the wrong time in the wrong way, its effects will be minimal or even negative. Of course, this is true of all medicines, but especially of the kingly Chinese remedies. In general, if the consumer is guided by the uses of ginseng suggested in this book, there will be little chance of any side effects.

CHAPTER 9

Balancing the Old
and the New

I t has taken literally thousands of years for
ginseng to appear in stores in the West. Doctors are not generally familiar with it, and
those who are often regard it as yet another useless fad.
The climate of medical opinion has hardly changed from
that put forward in the Smithsonian Institute report at the
beginning of this century: "Ginseng has no value as far as
Western medicine can judge . . . its effects being purely
psychological . . . but we have only scratched the surface
of Chinese medical knowledge."

Only a few years ago top medical experts of the West
were saying exactly the same thing about acupuncture: It
had no real value, it was mere trickery or hypnotism. They
were often so scathing in their condemnation that practitioners were hardly differentiated from witches. Now the
same experts have completely reversed their opinion, rec-
ognizing it as a technique of great potential usefulness,
even though medical experts in the West still do not understand how it works. It might be suggested that, like the
apparently paradoxical aspects of ginseng, it certainly will

be hard to understand any aspect of Chinese medicine if it is approached from a conventional point of view. It needs to be seen from the perspective of traditional medicine and the Chinese view of the body and its ailments.

UNDERSTANDING WESTERN PREJUDICES

It is quite possible that ginseng will follow the same road as acupuncture. One day it may be recognized as an important new aid to health and become not only widely used but widely accepted in the West. Meanwhile, the question might be raised: Why does the medical profession not take seriously such an obviously beneficial substance? Several reasons can be suggested.

First, many ginseng products made in Western countries are of such poor quality that the public and the medical profession both might have begun to be interested in ginseng when it arrived, only to dismiss it after trying various ginseng products with no apparent result.

Second, while as many as 2,000 reports have been published on ginseng in the scientific journals of China, Russia, Japan, and Korea, most of these have not been translated, and very few have been read by Western scientists. This is partly due to the difficulty of obtaining the articles, but mostly due to the indifference of Western experts to such information from the East. For the most part, the flow of medical and scientific knowledge has been in one direction—from West to East. Apart from an "information gap," there is also a "credibility gap." Even when information does arrive in the West, it is often ignored or treated with suspicion, for the experts trust neither the authors, whom they do not know, nor the journal, which they do not respect.

The third reason for Western medicine's dismissal of

ginseng is that Western medicines are mostly synthetic, and are strictly defined, manufactured, packaged, and distributed by a large pharmaceutical industry with a powerful voice in medicine. Doctors feel that unless a medicine is of this category, it should not be used. Their attitude has probably been formed by their medical school training and pharmaceutical industry advertising. The pharmaceutical industry is strongly opposed to natural medicines because it could not support itself on the distribution of herbs and roots.

Finally, ginseng, like many other herbs, has a mild and subtle effect, most beneficial when the root is taken regularly for some time. No specific disease can be said to be cured by ginseng. All of its effects are so different from conventional medicines that if compared with powerful synthetic drugs, ginseng may be regarded as inconsequential. Some features, such as its "adaptogenic" power, are puzzling if regarded from a conventional point of view, although they are well understood in traditional medicine. Therefore, ginseng has been thought about in the past in a way calculated to miss its most advantageous features.

SYNTHETIC DRUGS VERSUS HERBS

The strange fact is that although many doctors still do not think much of herbs and herbalism, a great many synthetic medicines these doctors use are originally derived from plants. They may have been extracted, altered, and resynthesized for the purpose of standardization and so on, but often the original discovery and isolation of the drug was based on traditional herbs. Digitalis, the important heart-stabilizing glycoside, came from the foxglove; morphine from the poppy; quinine, once vital in the treatment of malaria, from the bark of a tree; reserpine, used in the treatment of mental disease, from Rauwolfia root. The list is enormous. No one would deny that the pharmaceutical industry was founded on plants.

Perhaps it is not so widely known that much research is still being done to find more and more new medicines from traditional plant remedies. Not long ago, the powerful anticancer alkaloids vinblastine and vincristine were found in the plant *Vinca rosea*, used since ancient times in Indian medicine, while taxol, a brand new anticancer drug, is now being made from the yew tree, a traditional Western herbal medicine. The United States' multi-million-dollar drive against cancer includes a massive new survey of plants used in traditional medicine in an attempt to find new anticancer drugs.

It would thus be more accurate to say that the medical world is not opposed to plants as such, only to those that have not yet yielded chemically defined and standardized chemicals. As one eminent British scientist said about ginseng, "It is no use doing any research on it until we know what it contains." This attitude is precisely what prevents Western medical experts from understanding and utilizing the wealth of traditional medicines. Who cares what chemicals are in the plant, as long as it works safely? There is no point in forgetting the aims of medicine because of a habit of extracting and synthesizing drugs.

COMPONENTS ARE NOT ENOUGH

Besides ignoring some important medicines that happen to be too complicated to yield known active ingredients, Western doctors may be making another error. The process of extracting and defining the active components may leave out other constituents that are essential to balanced treatment.

The herbalist understands that medicines must be as subtly harmonized as music. Extraction of only one component is like throwing out all the instruments in an orchestra except the loudest. This may be harmful. For example, aspirin is acetyl salisylic acid, one of the many components of willow. It was extracted in the seventeenth century, probably the first medicine to be purified and synthesized. After 300 years of constant use, it has now been shown to cause side effects such as stomach bleeding. However, extracts of willow bark and the parent compounds from which aspirin is derived, especially the main one called salicin, are all known to be very safe and to cause no stomach damage. Therefore, it would have been better not to use aspirin in such a concentrated and purified form.

Ginseng is one of the few herbs about which there is clear scientific evidence that the whole plant has more medicinal powers than any of the chemicals so far isolated from it. Some day ginsenoside pills may be available at your local pharmacy. In both the Soviet Union and Japan, ginsenoside-rich extract is now made for the pharmaceutical industry from ginseng root material grown in vats in the laboratory. But because of the great number of constituents, many still unknown, it is obvious that a great deal will be lost when a ginsenoside pill is made.

Conventional scientific research, in attempting to extract a single chemical, also looks for a single defined action of a drug. For example, tests may be carried out to see if a drug can raise or lower blood pressure. Ginseng is perhaps unique as the first herb for which there is scientific evidence that the whole root can have multiple and apparently paradoxical effects. It can both raise and lower the blood pressure or act as both stimulant and sedative. Conventional medicine would prefer one defined drug to raise the blood pressure and another to lower it, but neither one could adjust to the body's requirements as ginseng does.

A HOPEFUL FUTURE

The very philosophy behind conventional medicine needs to be brought up to date. But it would be foolish to go to the opposite extreme and become prejudiced against conventional medicine. There are, of course, a multitude of things the more powerful synthetic medicines can do that herbs cannot. One need only think of the new drugs available that can now cure pneumonia, leprosy, and malaria; the vaccines that can completely protect against smallpox or polio; and the affordable insulin that can greatly prolong the life of diabetics while keeping them in relatively good health. The point is that there are gaps in conventional medicine that could be very successfully filled by natural medicine, and herbal treatment should be used alongside conventional medicine, as in China. Herbs should be used as safe treatment for mild common health problems or as restoratives and tonics to maintain health, while the stronger medicines should be used when a serious illness occurs despite all the other efforts, as mentioned in the Emperor Shen Nung's *Pharmacopoeia of the Heavenly Husbandman*. This would be the best of the old and the new.

Ginseng is being used a little more widely every day. It is already available in all health stores in the Western world and is the main constituent in several geriatric preparations for sale in pharmacies. We can expect that as it gets more widely known, serious research on its properties might begin in the West. Doctors might know more about it and prescribe courses of it to increase the health of their patients, as they already do in Russia and China.

In Britain and America, ginseng is not readily accepted by the medical profession. There is little chance that it will enter the English language pharmacopeias in the very near future. On the other hand, there are many enthusiasts who take ginseng, including some doctors and psychiatrists.

Henry Kissinger, who skipped around the world with such energy, made headlines when it was found that he carried ginseng. Many internationally known sportsmen, such as the world-record-breaking British athlete Sebastian Coe, take ginseng. During the long hours of the Paris peace conference on Vietnam, members of the North Vietnamese delegation never appeared to be tired or exhausted. When questioned about this by the other diplomats, they produced their ginseng with a flourish.

The last word should come from Sir Edwin Arnold, the famous traveler, translator, and author, who eloquently summed up the case for ginseng as a result of his experience in China.

> According to the Chinese, Asiatic ginseng is the best and most potent of all cordials, stimulants, tonics, stomachics, cardiacs, febrifuges, and above all, will best renovate and invigorate failing forces. It fills the heart with hilarity, while its occasional use will, it is said, add a decade to human life. Can all these generations of Orientals who have praised heaven for ginseng's many benefits have been totally deceived? Was humanity ever quite mistaken when half of it believed in something never puffed and never advertised?

Further Reading

Fulder, Stephen. *The Book of Ginseng, and Other Chinese Herbs for Vitality.* Healing Arts Books, Rochester, Vermont (1993).

Harding, A.R. *Ginseng and Other Medicinal Plants.* Facsimile of the original 1908 edition published by Emporium Publications, Boston, Mass. (1972).

Harriman, Sarah. *The Book of Ginseng.* Pyramid Books, New York (1975).

Kaptchuk, Ted. *The Web That Has No Weaver, Understanding Chinese Medicine.* St. Martins Press, New York (1984).

Korngold, Harriet. *Between Heaven and Earth: A Guide to Chinese Medicine.* Ballantine, New York (1991).

Mills, Simon. *Out of the Earth.* Viking Penguin, New York (1991).

Ody, Penelope. *The Herb Society's Complete Medicinal Herbal.* Dorling Kindersley, London (1993).

Pelletier, Kenneth. *Holistic Medicine: From Stress to Optimum Health.* Delta/Seymour Lawrence, New York (1990).

Teeguarden, Ron. *Chinese Tonic Herbs.* Japan Publications, Tokyo and New York (1984).

Tierra, Michael. *Planetary Herbology.* Lotus Press, Santa Fe, New Mexico (1992).

Useful Research Summaries

Baldwin, C.A., Anderson, L.A., and Phillipson, J.D. "What Pharmacists Should Know about Ginseng." *Pharmaceutical Journal,* 237, 583–586 (1986).

Brekhman, I.I. and Dardymov, I.V. "New Substances of Plant Origin Which Increase Nonspecific Resistance." *Annual Review of Pharmacology,* 9, 419–430 (1969).

Chong, S.K.F. and Oberholzer, V.G. "Ginseng—Is There a Use in Clinical Medicine?" *Postgraduate Medical Journal,* 64, 841–846 (1988).

Hallstrom, C., Fulder, S.,and Carruthers, M. "Effect of Ginseng on Performance of Nurses on Night Duty." *Comparative Medicine East and West,* 6, 277–282 (1982).

Lewis, W. "Ginseng: a Medical Enigma." In: Etkin, N.L., (ed.) *Plants in Indigenous Medicine & Diet: Biobehavioral Approaches.* Redgrave Publishing, Bedford Hills, New York (1986).

Liu, C-X, and Xiao, P-G. "Recent Advances on Ginseng Research in China." *Journal of Ethnopharmacology,* 36, 27–38 (1992).

Ng, T.B., and Yeun, H.W. "Scientific Basis of the Therapeutic Effects of Ginseng." In: Steiner, R. P. (Ed.) *Folk Medicine: The Art and the Science.* American Chemical Society, Washington (1986).

Owen, R, T. "Ginseng: a Pharmacological Profile." *Drugs of Today,* 18, 343–351 (1981).

Phillipson, J.D. and Anderson, L.A. "Ginseng—Quality, Safety and Efficacy?" *Pharmaceutical Journal*, 232, 161–165 (1984).

Shibata, S., et al. "Chemistry and Pharmacology of Panax." In: Wagner, H., Hikino, H., and Farnsworth, N.R., (Eds.) *Economic and Medicinal Plant Research* Vol. 1. Academic Press, London (1985).

Wicklund, I., Karlberg, J., and Lund, B. "A Double-Blind Comparison of the Effect on Quality of Life of a Combination of Vital Substances including Standardized Ginseng G115 and Placebo. *Current Therapeutic Research*, 55, 32–42 (1994).

INDEX